MEDICAL SCHOOL
FROM HIGH SCHOOL

MEDICAL SCHOOL FROM HIGH SCHOOL

THE COLLEGE APPLICANT'S
GUIDE TO MEDICAL SCHOOL
EARLY ADMISSION PROGRAMS

2ND EDITION

A. AZAM & A.M. ILYAS, MD

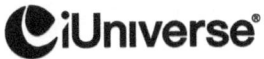

MEDICAL SCHOOL FROM HIGH SCHOOL
THE COLLEGE APPLICANT'S GUIDE TO MEDICAL SCHOOL EARLY ADMISSION PROGRAMS
2nd EDITION

The information, ideas, and suggestions in this book are not intended as a substitute for professional medical advice. Before following any suggestions contained in this book, you should consult your personal physician. Neither the author nor the publisher shall be liable or responsible for any loss or damage allegedly arising as a consequence of your use or application of any information or suggestions in this book.

iUniverse books may be ordered through booksellers or by contacting:

iUniverse
1663 Liberty Drive
Bloomington, IN 47403
www.iuniverse.com
1-800-Authors (1-800-288-4677)

Because of the dynamic nature of the Internet, any web addresses or links contained in this book may have changed since publication and may no longer be valid. The views expressed in this work are solely those of the author and do not necessarily reflect the views of the publisher, and the publisher hereby disclaims any responsibility for them.

Any people depicted in stock imagery provided by Thinkstock are models, and such images are being used for illustrative purposes only. Certain stock imagery © Thinkstock.

ISBN: 978-1-5320-0977-8 (sc)
ISBN: 978-1-5320-0978-5 (e)

Library of Congress Control Number: 2016918170

Print information available on the last page.

iUniverse rev. date: 12/21/2016

CONTENTS

Program Profiles

Undergraduate Institution   Medical Institution

Alabama

University of South Alabama University of South Alabama College
of Medicine

California

University of California,   University of California, Los Angeles
Riverside   School of Medicine

University of California, San University of California, San Diego
Diego   School of Medicine

Connecticut

University of Connecticut	University of Connecticut School of Medicine

Colorado

University of Colorado, Denver	University of Colorado Anshultz Medical Campus

District of Columbia

George Washington University (7–8 years)	George Washington University School of Medicine
St. Bonaventure University	George Washington University School of Medicine
Howard University	Howard University College of Medicine

Florida

University of Miami (7–8 years)	University of Miami School of Medicine

Hawaii

University of Hawaii, Manoa	University of Hawaii Johns A. Burns School of Medicine

Illinois

Northwestern University	Northwestern University Medical School

Indiana

Indiana State University	Indiana University School of Medicine

Kentucky

University of Kentucky	University of Kentucky College of Medicine

Massachusetts

Boston University	Boston University School of Medicine

Missouri

University of Missouri, Kansas City	University of Missouri, Kansas City School of Medicine

New Jersey

Caldwell University	Rutgers—New Jersey Medical School
The College of New Jersey	Rutgers—New Jersey Medical School
Drew University	Rutgers—New Jersey Medical School
Montclair State University	Rutgers—New Jersey Medical School
New Jersey Institute of Technology	Rutgers—New Jersey Medical School
Rutgers University, Newark	Rutgers—New Jersey Medical School
Stevens Institute of Technology	Rutgers—New Jersey Medical School

New Mexico

University of New Mexico	University of New Mexico School of Medicine

New York

Brooklyn College	State University of New York, Downstate Medical Center College of Medicine
Rensselaer Polytechnic Institute	Albany Medical College

University of Rochester	University of Rochester of Medicine and Dentistry
Sophie Davis School of Biomedical Education	City University of New York Medical School
State University of New York,	State University of New York, Stony Brook
Stony Brook	School of Medicine Health Science Center
Union College	Albany Medical College

North Carolina

East Carolina University	Brody School of Medicine at East Carolina University

Ohio

University of Akron	Northeastern Ohio Universities College of Medicine
Case Western Reserve University	Case Western Reserve University School of Medicine
University of Cincinnati	University of Cincinnati College of Medicine
Kent State University	Northeastern Ohio Universities College of Medicine
Miami University	University of Cincinnati College of Medicine
Youngstown State University	Northeastern Ohio Universities College of Medicine

Pennsylvania

Drexel University	Drexel University College of Medicine
Lehigh University	Drexel University College of Medicine
Monmouth University	Drexel University College of Medicine

Pennsylvania State University	Sydney Kimmel Medical College of Thomas Jefferson University
Rosemont College	Drexel University College of Medicine
Temple University	Temple University School of Medicine
University of Pittsburg	University of Pittsburg School of Medicine Drexel University College of Medicine
Ursinus College	
Villanova University	Drexel University College of Medicine
West Chester University	Drexel University College of Medicine
Widener University	Temple University School of Medicine
Wilkes University	SUNY, Upstate Medical University College of Medicine
Wilkes University	Pennsylvania State University College of Medicine

Rhode Island

Brown University	Warren Alpert Brown University School of Medicine

Texas

Rice University	Baylor College of Medicine
Texas A&M University	Texas A&M University College of Medicine

Virginia

Virginia Commonwealth University	Virginia Commonwealth University School of Medicine

FOREWORD

Since I published the first edition of this book in 2001, I have witnessed a boom in both the number and interest in medical school early-admission programs. Also during this time of great technological advancement, we have witnessed a change in the way students study, the way high schools educate, and the way colleges evaluate applicants. The SAT test has also changed significantly during this time. However, during this time, the interest and demand for medical school admissions remains high, thereby maintaining the value of this book.

To the best of our knowledge, this book continues to offer the most comprehensive listing of medical school early-admission programs.

ASIF M. ILYAS, MD, FACS
Associate Professor of Orthopedic Surgery
The Rothman Institute at the Thomas Jefferson University
Philadelphia, Pennsylvania

PREFACE

To practice medicine is perhaps one of the greatest privileges society can offer an individual. For this reason, it is not surprising that competition for medical school admission is perennially so great. However, medical school early-admission programs have continued to fly under the radar. These programs offer an enriching and expeditious route for committed high school students to pursue careers in medicine. It is my hope that, with this book, more individuals undaunted by hard work and committed to joining the admirable field of medicine may increase their chances of becoming physicians.

My own perspective comes not only from my personal experiences of applying and being accepted to multiple medical school early-admission programs but also from the experience I gained by advising my siblings, relatives, and friends into securing admission into these programs. Throughout the years, I have amassed a considerable database of information on these programs. In addition, while in medical school, I had the opportunity to act as a student admissions interviewer as well as a student ambassador. These experiences allowed me to understand the point of view of admissions personnel in addition to the student perspective.

Allow me to end this preface by saying that—along with my new partner and coauthor for this second edition, Aysha Azam—we have made every effort to be as diligent as possible in conveying the most accurate information to you, the reader. If there are any discrepancies, we strongly encourage you to contact me so changes can be made in future editions. In addition, I ask students, deans, and program advisers to contact me if there are any changes to the currently included programs, listed in part B, or if any new programs have been started so I can add them to future editions. I can be reached at aimd2001@ yahoo.com.

In short, I believe this book is a must-have for any high school student committed to a career in medicine and a mandatory reference book for every high school and college career guidance office in the country. If this resource helps even one college applicant committed to becoming a physician to gain admission to one of the many wonderful medical school early-admission programs, my time has been well spent.
—A. M. ILYAS, MD

PART A

CHAPTER 1

WHAT IS A MEDICAL SCHOOL EARLY-ADMISSION PROGRAM?

Medical school early-admission programs are programs for high school students who know they want to go to medical school. It simultaneously accepts students straight from high school to both an undergraduate college and a medical school. In this way, students begin college with acceptance to a medical school. These programs began to surface in the 1960s and were designed to give academically gifted and motivated high school students interested in medicine a fast track to becoming physicians. The motivation was to offset the period's decline in the number of available physicians, due to the war effort, as well as to address the decline in the number of applications to medical school. Decades later, these programs have prospered and grown in number. Yet during this period the number and quality of applications to medical schools has also grown.

Why have these programs persisted and even increased? The answer is that the experiment of accepting high school students preemptively to medical school resulted in other unforeseen benefits. It allowed local undergraduate and medical schools to recruit and keep intelligent, motivated, and dedicated students before potentially losing them to other competing institutions. It also provided an avenue to cultivate young minds more broadly by protecting them from the distraction of focusing on medical school admissions alone. These minds could now be free to contribute more to their communities, pursue more diverse research, or simply pursue other areas of study not otherwise possible for the traditional premedical student. In addition, some programs evolved to address particular needs of various geographic locales, especially the shortage of primary care physicians in rural areas.

What's the benefit?

Traditionally, to go to medical school, students had to graduate from high school, go to college, take the MCAT, and apply to medical school during their junior year of college. This avenue represents the vast majority of applications to medical school, generally resulting in approximately five hundred thousand applications annually, competing for a seat in the country's 141 medical schools.

In recent years, the acceptance rate overall for matriculation from undergraduate to medical school is 2.91 percent, per the Association of American Medical Colleges. Subsequently, the benefit of applying to a medical school early-admission program is competing within a considerably smaller applicant pool of other high school students. Another major benefit of early admission is the decreased level of stress and anxiety once enrolled through your college career; thereby allowing you to maximize your college experience.

How does it work?

The nuances of the application process will be detailed in chapter 3, "Understanding the Application Process." Moreover, each medical school early-admission program has individual requirements that are also outlined in detail in part B of the book, "Program Profiles." In short, applicants apply to the individual undergraduate institution sponsoring a program as seniors in high school (note: a few programs allow their students to apply after they are college freshmen or sophomores). If they meet the program's requirements for SAT scores, GPA, rank, and extracurricular activities (all of which will also be discussed in detail in later chapters), they will be invited for a formal interview.

Once accepted into a program, the student will spend between two to four years at the undergraduate institution—depending on the specific design of that program—before moving on to the participating medical school. While in college, the students will have to maintain a minimum GPA and participate in various enrichment programs, and they may be required to achieve a minimum score on the MCAT. Again, all of the specifics of each program are outlined in part B of this book.

Knowledge and effort are everything.

Before we go any further, allow us to define the most important underlying principle of how to successfully achieve acceptance to a medical school early-admission program or any professional aspiration in general, for that matter: Success does not lie in being the smartest. It lies in being the hardest working and the most informed.

There are countless stories of students who were exceptionally intelligent but lacked either the motivation to work hard or the correct information to guide them. Clearly, since you are reading this book, you are taking the first step toward being informed. As long as you add the second ingredient of hard work as well as the absolute prerequisite of an unwavering commitment to becoming a physician, then join us as we discuss the specifics of getting you into medical school from high school.

CHAPTER 2

MEDICAL SCHOOL EARLY-ADMISSION Q&AS

To help you understand early-admission medical programs, this chapter will answer some common questions we have encountered over the years.

How do medical school early-admission programs work?

Applying to medical school early-admission programs is no different than applying to colleges traditionally. The process particulars will be discussed in more detail in chapter 3: "Understanding the Application Process." In short, during the senior year of high school, applicants will submit standard undergraduate (college) applications, but applicants will note that they are applying to the college's medical school early-admission program.

Some programs may require additional forms and supporting documents. These requirements may include essays, additional letters of recommendation, SAT II scores, and/or details of extracurricular activities. If deemed a good candidate for the program by the college, the applicant will be invited to attend an interview session at the participating medical school. The interview will focus on assessing the applicant's commitment and potential to becoming a physician—as well as evaluating his or her academic ability, personal character, and maturity.

Once accepted into an early-admission program, students will begin their education in an undergraduate college. The number of years and credits needed to participate and complete in college will vary from program to program. Generally, the undergraduate duration of the program will consist of two to four years. During these undergraduate years, students will fulfill the general requirements of their majors.

However, students may have additional requirements, such as maintaining a minimum GPA and/or achieving a minimum MCAT score. In addition, early-admission students are awarded special benefits. In additional to the priceless peace of mind that comes from knowing they hold a seat in medical school, the students typically participate in various enrichment courses geared to preparing them for a career in medicine.

Following the completion of the assigned number of undergraduate years and/or credits and meeting the minimum GPA and/or MCAT requirements, students will be promoted to the participating medical school. Once matriculated into the medical school, the requirements as an early-admission student will be no different from those of any other medical student. The length of the medical school portion will be the standard four years, after which they will be awarded their medical degrees.

What's in it for me?

Applying from high school allows you to avoid competing with the approximately five hundred thousand premedical students applying to medical school from college on a yearly basis. Therefore, although applying for fewer available medical school early-admission program seats, applicants will now be competing within a much smaller and more select applicant pool.

Once accepted into an early-admission program, the greatest benefit is the peace of mind and educational freedom. For those who are unaware, the premedical student's undergraduate career is an extremely competitive, rigorous, anxiety-provoking, and often overwhelming time. Early-admission students avoid the stress and heartache of traditional medical school admissions, which allows them the time to pursue their own academic, research, and extracurricular pursuits. In addition, medical school early-admission programs generally sponsor various experiences to help prepare students for careers in medicine. Such experiences include working with physicians of various specialties, health-outreach programs, and participating in medical research while still in college.

Moreover, some students also gain other benefits by enrolling in an early-admission medical program. Depending on the college, one such benefit is being admitted into the college's honors program, which carries its own perks. These include being able to take special or limited-enrollment courses, scheduling classes before other students (priority scheduling), and access to special housing accommodations.

Though all of these benefits are great, one of the greatest benefits of the medical school early-admission program can be financial. Accepted students tend to receive significant financial rewards and recognitions in the form of merit-based scholarships and grants. Scholarship money is among a college's greatest tools for luring the most qualified applicants to enroll in their institution. Of course, the amount of the scholarships or grants varies based on the college.

Should I pass on an Ivy League college?

This is a very personal decision, and there is no right or wrong answer. Most medical school early-admission programs are not linked with Ivy League or more "prestigious" colleges. Oftentimes, the high school students who are competitive enough to secure acceptance to a medical school early-admission program can also secure acceptance to more prestigious colleges. However, getting accepted to medical school is quite difficult regardless of the prestige and reputation of your college. There are some things to consider when determining whether to go to medical school through an early-admission program or go the more traditional route by attending a prestigious college.

Prestige offers a number of advantages, including the weight of the institution's name, resources, and legacy. Being part of this legacy provides a strong "network" or "connections" that can help a premedical applicant. In addition, prestigious institutions offer greater resources and quality of coursework, research, and extracurricular opportunities.

However, disadvantages of applying from a more prestigious college as a premedical student exist as well. Competition among the premedical students at a prestigious college can be fiercer. Other students will be equally intelligent and motivated to excel and compete. They will be competing for a limited number of A's, for the attention of the faculty, good letters of recommendation, and the most exciting research opportunities.

On the road to becoming a physician, college is just another step; it is not the final step. These steps include high school, college, medical school, and residency. When choosing a college, it is important to consider its prestige and how it will impact the ultimate goal of becoming a physician.

Can I change my mind about being a doctor after I've started?

Yes, you can change your mind after starting the program while in college.

Am I sacrificing the length of my undergraduate experience?

Medical school early-admission programs come in various lengths. Certain programs are accelerated, and you will spend only two or three years in college. Other programs incorporate a full unaccelerated four years of college. In addition, programs vary in the number of credits that a student has to complete before being promoted to medical school. In short, programs come in various shapes and forms. Each is tailored to fit a particular mold designed to meet the program's goals. As an applicant, you choose the program that best fits your needs and wishes.

Will I still have a well-rounded undergraduate experience?

Definitely—and likely more so. You will have the time and the peace of mind to venture out, try different things, and participate in activities and organizations that you might not otherwise have had the freedom from your premedical studies to do so. Also, you will see as you read part B, "Program Profiles," that most programs provide and encourage their students to participate in various enrichment experiences meant to challenge and prepare them for careers in medicine.

Are these programs right for me?

Again, this is a very personal question. We have tried to highlight commonly asked questions about medical school early-admission programs through a simulated question-and-answer session. However, this discussion assumes the underlying premise that you are committed to a career in medicine. If you are unsure about becoming a physician, these programs may not be right for you.

For those still committed to attaining acceptance into medical school early-admission programs, let's continue our discussion and delve into the details of the application process.

CHAPTER 3

UNDERSTANDING THE APPLICATION PROCESS

Applying for a medical school early-admission program is initially the same as applying to a college. However, those high school students dedicated to becoming physicians and wanting an assured admission to a medical school from high school must begin their preparation much earlier than their senior year of high school. If you're reading this book, you are clearly motivated and well on your way to achieving your goal!

Through the Admission Officer's Eyes

For you to optimize your efforts, you must first understand what admissions officers are looking for when they look at your application. Even if you consider certain aspects of your application to be the strongest points, the officer may review your application with different priorities in mind. For that reason, the best way to ensure that you have a competitive application is for you to see your application as the admissions officer would. The general order of importance of high school credentials from the point of view of an admissions officer is:

(1) SAT
(2) GPA/Rank
(3) interview
(4) extracurricular activities (school, community, and medical)

Please do not be disheartened or discouraged by the order in this list; inevitably, some things on this list may be stronger than others. We will elaborate on the details of each and explain why they are where they are on this list. The underlying premise is that understanding the importance of your various credentials can be the vital difference that distinguishes an average applicant from a shoe-in applicant. With this information, you can concentrate your energy where it counts most and maximize your credentials and their presentation in a manner to optimize your application.

SAT? What about my grades?

It may come as a shock to hear that a high SAT score is more important than a good GPA—even if your teachers and guidance counselors have been telling you otherwise. The SAT is extremely important for a number of reasons. First, many admissions officers use these numbers as the primary cutoffs to decide which of the hundreds of applications to evaluate further. Second, the SAT is a standardized exam. Therefore, every applicant takes the same exam, under the same conditions, and is graded on the same scale. The scores on these tests give the best indication of how you match up against your peers regardless of other more subjective variables, such as your grades, your appearance, your school, or your athletic accomplishments. Third, the SAT tests show how you prepare for and handle high-stress situations. For many high school students, this test is the first big challenge. How you prepare and respond to it says volumes about your potential to succeed in medical school and your professional life in general.

What do you mean my grades are subjective?

After your SAT scores, your high school GPA and class rank are second on the list of important credentials. They are second because of their inherent subjectivity. High school grades are subjective due to variations in coursework difficulty, instruction, grading, and peer competition between schools, regions, states, etc. Therefore, unlike the SAT, which is the same for everyone, how hard it was for you to get an A in sophomore year chemistry can vary significantly, depending on which high school you attend. In defense of every teacher who has pushed us to work hard at our grades, getting an A is always important no matter where you go to school—and it is expected if you plan to go on to medical school.

Interview? What do I talk about?

We will discuss the ins and outs of the medical school interview in detail in chapter 6. As a high school student, your medical school early-admission program interview will probably be your first "professional" interview. Generally, applicants applying to colleges do not have to interview. However, all medical school admissions require interviews. At this junction, we leave you with three words to think about until we arrive at chapter 6: *confidence, maturity,* and *commitment.* You must convey these attributes during your interview.

Should I volunteer at a local hospital?

Absolutely! Volunteering and demonstrating a genuine interest in medicine is very important. Once your SAT scores and grades land you an interview, your extracurricular activities will help the admissions officer get a better sense of who you are personally. Subsequently, the extracurricular activities you choose—both in school as well as outside of school, like at the local hospital or organizations for the needy—allow you to paint the picture you want of yourself. Moreover, during the interview, these activities will provide you with material to discuss about yourself.

Let's discuss this in more detail.

The activities you pursue in your community will be strongly scrutinized. Admissions officers will look for a commitment to community service, involvement in health care–related activities, and participation in leadership roles. They seek these virtues because these are the virtues that society seeks in physicians.

Don't quit your mall job, but do also consider working as a camp counselor or volunteering in a local medical clinic or nursing home. These activities are mutually beneficial. It allows you to contribute to your community in a tangible manner while allowing you to learn more about real-life medicine. Other community service suggestions include training as an EMT, volunteering in an ER, learning/teaching CPR, and supporting the Red Cross.

What about the school play?

Participating in service-related extracurricular activities outside of school does not mean that you should ignore extracurricular activities in school (sports, clubs, drama, etc.). What you actually do and the amount of time you ultimately commit to these activities is not always the priority of admissions officers. Admissions officers want to see committed, well-rounded students who demonstrate time-management skills. Participating in extracurricular activities is a great way to be a part of your school community. It is a healthy and productive outlet for your energy, abilities, and talents. It is a way to express your intellectual, organizational, and social skills. It is a way to make friends, contact members of the community, and get to know your school faculty. And, at the very least, it is fun.

Sports, just as school clubs, can illustrate how well-rounded you are. School sports, however, can provide an added advantage if you are a recognized athlete in a particular sport with scholarships. Another benefit is the opportunity to interview with an individual who shares the same enthusiasm for a sport. These are wonderful circumstances that can make your application stand out and provide opportunities to personally relate with your interviewer.

School clubs, particularly nationally recognized ones, are excellent organizations in which to be involved. Similarly, participating in student government provides an applicant with the opportunity to be a class leader and an avenue to be recognized by school faculty and administration. Honor societies are also excellent organizations in which to be involved in, particularly since membership requires meeting certain academic criteria. These honors inherently distinguish you from the rest of your class. Honor society membership also demonstrates that an applicant is a competitive and active student at the school and on a national level.

Extracurricular activities, including school sports, clubs, and community activities, are vital to a well-rounded application. However, we will leave you with one warning: participating in activities should never occur at the expense of your grades. Remember, poor grades means no interview. Time management will be key in maintaining good grades and pursuing your extracurricular interests.

The Main Course

Allow us to leave you with this metaphor: consider your application as a meal being served to an admissions officer at a restaurant. Your SAT and GPA/rank are the main course. Your extracurricular activities are the condiments, and your interview is the quality of service. Without a good main course, the condiments and service are irrelevant. However, with bad service (a poor interview), even a good main course may not be enjoyable.

CHAPTER 4

THE SATS

SAT is the well-known acronym for the Scholastic Assessment Test. It is more specifically known as the SAT I—the Reasoning Test, and it also affectionately known as the College Board—named after the nonprofit organization that has been administering the exam for more than a hundred years. (There is also the SAT II—the Subject Tests, which will be discussed shortly).

The SAT I is a three-hour-and-forty-five-minute test consisting of:

- four critical reading sections: three twenty-five-minute sections and one twenty-minute section
- four math sections: three twenty-five-minute sections and one twenty-minute section
- two writing sections: one twenty-five-minute sections and one ten-minute section

The verbal questions are designed to test your ability to understand and analyze what you read, recognize relationships between parts of a sentence, and establish relationships between pairs of words. The math questions are designed to test your abilities in arithmetic, algebra, geometry, statistics, and probability. The writing questions are designed to test your ability to identify sentence errors, improve sentences, and improve paragraphs. It also comprises an essay portion (included in the writing section) that will test your writing abilities.

The SAT is scored out of a maximum of 2400. The verbal, math, and writing sections count for a maximum score of 800 each. Test takers start with a minimum score of 200 on each section. Therefore, potential scores can range from 600 to 2400 points.

For more logistical specifics on the SAT, refer to the College Board website: http://sat.collegeboard.org/home

It's just one test!

It is true that the SAT is only one exam. However, the reality is that it can define a student academically. The reason is simple: it serves as the one true objective performance measure available to admissions officers. As discussed earlier, even though you spend every day working on your high school records, all of your grades are influenced by a certain degree of inherent subjectivity. Variations abound between differences in high school coursework difficulty, instruction, grading, and peer competition. The SAT controls for all that. The same exam is offered to every student, with the same level of difficulty, under the same conditions, and graded in the same way. In addition to its objectivity, it also reflects how students prepare for and respond to a single stressful situation.

The SAT, the SAT, and the SAT

If someone asked us about the three most important credentials in your application to a medical school early-admission program, we would reply, "First, the SAT, second, the SAT, and third, the SAT." It is unfortunate that a single exam carries so much weight, but as we discussed earlier, it is the single most objective representation of a student's ability. Don't be confused by this statement. The SAT's extreme importance stems from its objective characteristics and its common use as the primary weeding tool for determining who is interviewed and who is not. However, admission to medical school cannot be secured without the other application components, such as grades and extracurricular activities.

Just the beginning of a long line of tests.

There is another nuance to the SAT as it relates to the field of medicine. Another reason why the SAT is weighed so heavily when considering students to medical school early-admission programs is because the SAT is just the first in a long line of standardized tests that that a student aspiring to become a physician will have to take. The SAT is followed by the MCAT in college.

In medical school, there is the United States Medical Licensing Exam (USMLE) Step 1 exam during the second year and the USMLE Step 2 exam prior to graduation. In residency, there will be the USMLE Step 3. Upon completing residency, there will be your specialty's board certification exam. Then, as a practicing physician, there are license-renewing exams every few years.

Successful standardized test-taking ability is important for medical school applicants due to the regular testing demands in the medical field. A student's performance on the SAT exam represents his or her current ability and preparedness, and it serves as a yardstick for predicting future performance on standardized exams.

When should I take the SAT?

High schools generally recommend taking the SAT during junior year and during the first semester of the senior year (if necessary). Technically, there is no limit to when and how often you can take the exam. Although the exam can be taken more than once, taking it more than three times is frowned upon and often not feasible due to time constraints. Since most students take the SAT for the first time during junior year, preparation must begin well in advance. A good time to commence preparation is the summer between sophomore and junior year (after receiving PSAT scores).

The PSAT

In order to begin mapping out your SAT preparation, it is important to gauge one's baseline ability on the SAT for diagnostic purposes. One such opportunity is to take the PSAT during sophomore year of high school. The PSAT is the acronym for the Preliminary Scholastic Aptitude Test. It serves two purposes: to provide a run through and preview of the SAT and to provide a platform for students to qualify for various scholarship and recognition programs, sponsored by the National Merit Scholarship Corporation. The PSAT is an abridged form of the SAT I and is designed to measure a student's critical-reading, math problem-solving, and writing abilities. It is scored out of 240, with a maximum score of 80 on the critical reading, math, and writing sections. Thus the PSAT is based on one-tenth of the scoring scale of the SAT I.

The PSAT, which is considered for scholarship purposes, is the one offered in the fall of a student's junior year. A great way to begin preparation for the SAT is by taking the PSAT during the sophomore year with the current juniors. It can serve as a diagnostic test and provide information on your baseline ability under standardized conditions. It will also define how much work you have ahead of you.

SAT Preparation Suggestions

Many resources are available for those seeking help with SAT preparation. Before mentioning some of the test preparation sources, allow us to share a few test taking tips to help improve your score.

Questions, questions, questions: The quickest way to improve your score on the SAT, and on other standardized exams for that matter, is to do lots and lots of questions. Practicing a high volume of questions has multiple benefits: Reviewing the answers to questions in detail helps you understand the question-writer's logic and thought processes, which will permeate through future questions. It introduces you to commonly tested themes. It improves your timing and endurance. Lastly, it will decrease anxiety by increasing your familiarity and comfort level with the exam in general.

Time management: Be conscious of the amount of time you spend on each question and the amount allotted to you for each section. Wear a watch during the exam. Do not spend too much time on any single question. Overall, the best way to improve your endurance and time management, or your speed in answering questions is, again, by doing a lot of questions.

Avoid omitting: The SAT is one of the few exams you will encounter that actually penalizes you for getting the wrong answer. Specifically, you are penalized a quarter point. Therefore, guessing is formally discouraged. In reality, this penalization often results in a stigma where students are afraid to make educated guesses and causes them to believe that omitting is probably better than guessing. This is absolutely false. We are not suggesting that you guess at every question you are unsure of, but we are recommending that if you can rule out at least one or two question choices, then make an educated guess. The benefit of guessing correctly in one out of every four guesses will improve your score more than just omitting four questions. If you have absolutely no idea on a question, it is probably better to omit. If you can rule out one or two options, it is often worth taking an educated guess. Again, doing a large volume of practice questions will help refine your skills in the process of elimination and the cost/benefit of omitting questions.

SAT Preparatory Resources

A slew of resources are available for SAT preparation. They vary considerably in price as well as in quality. Many classes and books are available, and each has its pros and cons. Below are listed some well-respected resources. Remember that many more qualified programs do exist. Also, remember that what works for some may not work for others.

Determining which resource you would like to use, if any, depends on your own style of studying and learning needs. It is always a good idea to ask around, especially senior students, to see what worked for them. Books are always cheaper than courses. Courses typically run upward of $2,000, which is a hefty sum of money. But, in the grand scheme, compared to the amount of money you will commit to your undergraduate and medical education, the amount you spend on test preparation is just a drop in the bucket. At minimum, seek a good bank of practice questions. Question banks are available from test prep courses, and many books geared toward SAT preparation are available in bookstores.

Below is a listing of some common test-prep courses and resources:

The College Boards	http: //www.collegeboards.org/
Kaplan	http: //www.kaplan.com/
Princeton Review	http: //www.princetonreview.com/
Scholastic Testing Service	http: //www.testprep.com/
College Power Prep	http: //www.powerprep.com/
Barron's	http: //www.barronseduc.com/
Peterson's	http: //www.petersons.com/

The SAT II

The SAT IIs are subject tests. They are a collection of one-hour exams covering a variety of subjects, including literature, US history, world history, mathematics, biology, chemistry, physics, and a variety of foreign languages. The individual subject exams are one hour long, and you can take up to three subject exams on one exam date. Each subject exam is scored out of a maximum score of 800. Again, preparation is necessary to excel on these exams. Good resources to use include the ones listed earlier. Preparation is even more critical for these since they test your factual knowledge on a specific topic—not just your reasoning abilities as in the SAT I. On the same token, it may be easier to prepare for these because they are topic-specific tests. As a rule of thumb, it is better to concern yourself with preparation for the SAT II after you have prepared for and successfully taken the SAT I. Dividing your time between preparations for both exams can prove counterproductive.

Many colleges require or recommend taking two or more of the SAT II subject tests for admission or placement. A variety of medical school early-admission programs require SAT II subject tests. The majority of schools recommend taking the biology, chemistry, or physics SAT II. Please refer to part B for specific SAT II requirements for the different programs.

CHAPTER 5

GPA/RANK

Your GPA and class rank are the summation of your academic career in high school. Although senior year grades also may come into play, college applications generally reflect grades through the junior year when initially submitted. The importance of attaining good grades goes without saying. Therefore, we won't bore you with mundane slogans like just do your best. Rather, let us discuss what medical school early-admission programs are looking for in particular.

As and Bs, right?

Many of the medical school early-admission programs have specific requirements for high school grades, ranging from a minimum GPA of 3.5 to some that require a 4.0 in order to be considered. Since GPA requirements vary, just assume "the higher, the better." You should at minimum expect to maintain a 3.5 to 4.0, or at least a 90 percent.

As for rank, not every program considers a student's class rank. For those that do, rank requirements vary from requiring a student to rank in the top 25 percent to the top 5 percent of their high school classes. However, admissions officers are aware that some high schools do not rank their students. Therefore, they will consider your GPA alone in its place.

Honors, Gifted, and AP Courses

Many high schools offer courses that are weighted heavier than others due to higher levels of difficulty or special enrollment requirements. Common examples of these courses include honors, gifted, or advanced placement (AP) courses. In certain schools, these courses may be weighted with additional bonus points to be added to the earned grade when calculating the GPA. Whether or not a course is weighted must be determined at the individual high school registrar's office.

In addition to the advantage of their weighted status, such honors courses also reflect positively on your transcript. Admission officers are keen at determining the difficulty of a student's high school course load. For example, they can appreciate the strength of a student who has earned a 3.5 GPA taking predominantly taking honors or AP courses versus a student who has a 3.9 GPA in all average to below average difficulty-level courses.

A word of warning: taking a weighted course may help bolster your GPA with additional points, but the courses are also generally more difficult. If you earn lower grades in these courses, taking them may outweigh the benefits. In addition, the grade that will appear on your transcript will be the unweighted one. Therefore, when considering weighted courses, remember that it is always better to get an "A" in a regular course than a "C" in a very difficult course. Be wise and carefully select your courses by assessing the intensity and considering your own ability and time. The best combination is taking all college-preparatory-caliber courses with some weighted courses sprinkled in which you are confident that you can do well in.

Strategies for Maximizing Your Grades

Review old questions/exams: As mentioned earlier in the discussion of the SAT, the best preparation is always to do a lot of questions. That goes for your coursework as well. Some teachers will provide old tests for review. For those who do not, senior students are a good resource for old exams. Old exam questions are an invaluable asset. Unfortunately, if a teacher does not want you to see an old exam, he/she won't allow students to keep them. The premise of this type of review is simple. It allows you to familiarize yourself with the subject matter and the teacher's style of questioning. As you will quickly see, the themes that a teacher wishes to stress do not vary much from year to year.

Understand, don't memorize: Understanding a concept is always more valuable than memorizing facts. Memorizing is generally considered to be the lowest form of learning. There is a place for it, however. Everyone must memorize certain things, especially doctors. However, whenever given the opportunity to learn something conceptually or theoretically, it is always worth your while to learn it conceptually. We always retain concepts better than random facts.

Make your own notes / flash cards: Most students study from a combination of a book and class notes. Making your own notes that highlight and review important points stressed in the book and class provide two major advantages. First, it provides a quick source of review material written in your own words and with your own understanding of the subject matter. Your own thoughts are generally better recollected than the thoughts of others. Second, it provides an exercise in physically writing down facts. Writing down or reiterating things is a form of reinforcement that can help you remember facts.

Study alone: Group studying, although fun, is often unproductive. Don't fall into the trap of studying in a group because of the theory that discussing and explaining a topic to one another allows you to understand it better. It is true that teaching someone can help fortify your own understanding as well as illustrate your grasp of a topic, but the premise relies on the notion that you have actually learned the material prior to a discussion. Initially, it is best to learn a topic conceptually on your own—without the distractions of a social forum.

Have fun: Remember the idiom, "All work and no play ..." Working hard in high school—and in college and medical school for that matter—requires a balance between work and leisure/personal/social time. You will always be more productive if you are happy, rested, and have some nonacademic interests to pursue.

CHAPTER 6

THE INTERVIEW

Almost every medical school early-admission program requires an interview. If you have been requested to appear for an interview, this means you have met all or most of a program's initial screening requirements (i.e., SAT and grades) and have moved on to the next round. All applicants invited for an interview are generally on equal footing. Interview performance coupled with credentials will dictate who will ultimately receive an offer for admission. As a general rule of thumb, programs interview two to four times as many applicants as there are seats available.

As a high school student, this will most likely be your first professional interview. Interviews can be a scary and intimidating experience for any person, regardless of age. However, preparation is key. Knowing what to expect and understanding what the interviewer wants will help relieve any associated anxiety as well as maximize the quality of the interview encounter.

Preparation and Practice

Allow me to preface this discussion on interviews by saying that not all good interviewees are "naturals." Rather, being able to interview well is an acquired trait that requires some preparation and practice. If you have reached the point of receiving an invitation to interview for a seat in a medical school early-admission program, you definitely have reason to develop your interviewing abilities.

Just as the SAT is the first in a long line of standardized exams, this interview will likely be the first in a long line of interviews on your road to becoming a physician. Therefore, prepare for your interviews seriously. Figure out what you want to show the interviewer and answer the questions accordingly. Practice answering the questions in an articulate and confident manner that demonstrates preparation and maturity. Mock interviews are a must, and they will give you the necessary practice to get you comfortable with your answers and the interview exchange in general. Like anything, the more you practice, the more at ease you will become.

Know where you are interviewing.

The first step in preparing for an interview is knowing all the players and places involved. You need to know as many details about the specific program, know the relevant facts about the participating college and medical school, and be familiar with the professional background of your interviewers. For instance, it would be embarrassing to begin an interview and not know whether the program is an accelerated six-year program or a full eight-year program. On the same token, it is a faux pas to address your interviewer as "Mr." or "Mrs." when they may more likely be "Dean," "Professor," or "Dr."

What will I say?

Although it is impossible and impractical to have a prepared answer for every question, it is reasonable to be prepared to answer some common questions or scenarios. For example, here are some commonly asked questions:

- Tell me about yourself.
- Tell me about your family.
- When did you first decide you wanted to become a doctor?
- How did you come to the decision that medicine is for you?
- Was there a single experience that led you to the decision to become a doctor?
- What specialty of medicine would you like to practice?
- Do you see yourself as a primary care doctor or a specialist?
- What do you like to do in your free time?
- What is your favorite sport?

- What is the last book you read?
- Who is your favorite author?
- What do you believe is your greatest strength?
- What do you believe is your greatest weakness?
- What do you believe has been your greatest achievement to this point?
- What do you believe has been your greatest failure to this point?
- What is the most difficult decision you have ever had to make?
- What leadership positions have you held?
- What was your favorite class?
- Who was your favorite teacher and why?
- Who has had the greatest impact on you?
- Where do you see yourself professionally in twenty years?
- Tell me something about yourself that separates you from the other applicants.

The above interview questions are some common general medical school interview questions. There are certain questions you will likely receive that are specific to the medical school early-admission program that you are interviewing for. They may include questions like:

- What leadership roles have you assumed?
- How did you come to the decision you wanted to be a doctor?
- Why are you interested in early admission to medical school?
- Why do you want to cut years off of your college experience?
- What features attract you to our program?
- How will you benefit from an early-admission medical school program?
- Do your parents want you to be a doctor?
- What hospital/medical-related experience have you had?
- How do you feel about working with sick and dying patients?
- Have you ever seen someone die?
- If you do not gain early admission to medical school, what will you do?
- What can you contribute to our program/institution?

These are just a handful of questions that you may be asked. The point is not to have specific answers to every question, but rather be prepared to answer questions regarding the root of your interest in medicine, your future practice ambitions, details about personal experiences mentioned on your application, and what qualities and strengths you have to offer. At first, it is hard to talk about oneself because it can feel unnatural under normal circumstances. An interview, however, is not a normal circumstance. It has its own rules, and one of those rules is to share your strengths and qualities freely and earnestly.

In addition to preparation for questions such as those posed above, be prepared to discuss various current events. Interviewers will not be expecting detailed summaries of the latest international peace accords, but they may be curious to see how well read and aware you are of such matters. In addition, health-related topics are always popular. For example, common topics include:

- Do you believe doctors make too much money?
- Is health care a right?
- How could we improve our nation's current health care disparities?
- How would you improve the organ donation process?
- How involved do you believe the government should be in health care?
- Do you believe abortion is a woman's right?
- What are your thoughts on euthanasia?
- What do you believe is America's role in helping foreign countries in need?
- Do you think the president/government is doing a good job with health care?

You may be thinking that these are tough and controversial questions, and you are right! These are tough questions because there is not always a right or wrong answer, and it may force you to take an unpopular position or at least one different from the interviewer. However, the goals of an interviewer with these controversial or difficult questions are to determine three things:

- Are you familiar and prepared to discuss the topic?
- Are you able to formulate an argument and support it?
- Are you able to respond under pressure?

The interviewer is not necessarily concerned with your particular opinion; instead, can you formulate and support your opinion while maintaining poise? One caveat: avoid expressing personal positions rooted in religion or politics. An interview for medical school is no time to be professing religious or partisan beliefs.

Beyond difficult or controversial questions, be prepared for curveball questions that are intended to throw you off balance. Interviewers have been known to say, "Let's see who can do more push-ups." Others may say, "Tell me a joke." Again, these questions are geared to see how you respond. Stay calm and maintain your poise.

Also, be prepared to answer questions about your résumé. The interviewer will have a copy of your extracurricular activities and areas of involvement. The interviewer can very reasonably ask you to elaborate on your participation in an extracurricular activity—from leadership roles to membership in an organization. Be sure to know the details of those activities to answer any questions. They can readily tell how involved or informed you are about your activities based on your comfort level discussing them.

What should I wear?

When you walk in to the office for the interview, you want to exude confidence and professionalism—and that starts with your appearance. Men should wear a navy blue or black contemporary-cut suit, a starched, clean dress shirt, and a subdued but fashionable tie. Women should wear a conservative suit or dress. Again, navy blue or black is best. Keep the dress length at or below the knees. Although a male interviewer may enjoy you wearing a provocative outfit, a female interviewer will not.

This also goes for excessive makeup. Both sexes should appear polished and groomed. Your clothing should be clean and free of wrinkles. Avoid excessive piercings. Men should avoid growing a beard or mustache during the interview period—and avoid trying out a new trendy haircut. If you already have a beard, make sure it is trimmed. Avoid anything flashy. This is not the time to show off your trendy wardrobe.

What else should I bring?

Aside from your sharp clothes, you should bring some paperwork. Specifically, bring a few copies of your resume that includes your name, contact information, high school information, SAT/grades/ rank, honors achieved, leadership positions, extracurricular activities, and employment information. In addition, bring a copy of your high school transcript with the latest grades and any recent achievements that may have occurred since the application was submitted. If you happened to have published something, bring a copy of the publication. In short, bring your resume (as a summary and reminder of yourself for the interviewer) and other things that illustrate your academic and leadership prowess or pertain to you professionally.

What do they want to see?

The personality traits that an interviewer wants to see immediately and throughout the interview can be summed up in three words: *confidence, maturity,* and *commitment.*

Confidence

Can you show that you are confident in yourself while being pleasant and affable—but not cocky? You must display a sense of self-assurance when you talk about yourself and answer their questions. However, you must remain pleasant and even and not get too aggressive or excited. Your confidence may be tested with the discussion of controversial topics. Again, the interviewer will not be concerned with your particular beliefs. Rather, he or she will want to observe your poise and ability to defend your positions. He or she wants to see that you have confidence in yourself and in your career goals. Show that you believe in yourself and what you can achieve.

Maturity

Can you hold an intellectual conversation with an older, daunting professional without being intimidated? Can you handle yourself in a foreign environment with poise? Can you discuss a topic, handle criticism, and support a stance without being too rigid or too agreeable? These are the subtle markers of maturity.

Commitment

Do you convey an unrelenting passion and commitment to pursuing a career in medicine? The slightest hint of being unsure about becoming a physician will be the kiss of death. They are deciding whether to make a huge commitment to you, and they need to know beyond a shadow of a doubt that you wish to be a doctor above all else.

Make sure that your résumé reflects your commitment to the medical field. For example, show dedication by volunteering at hospitals, shadowing doctors for an extended amount of time, or find a position as a research assistant with a professor in a lab. Conduct these activities during the summer or for another extended amount of time to show that you know what the medical field is like. This will also help when answering questions about current events. Show that you know what the medical field entails and that you are fully committed to it.

What should I do at the end?

At the end of the interview, you will be asked if you have any questions. The answer is an enthusiastic "Yes!" Asking questions when prompted displays your interest as well as preparedness. Have three to four intelligent questions ready. Again, be mindful of what you say. Do not ask any questions that may be construed as derogatory to the program, the institution, or any competitors. Also, do not ask any questions that may be inappropriate for the particular interviewer. For example, do not ask the chairperson of the department or program about the easiest way to get home. Save any logistical questions for the interview-day coordinator. Instead, ask appropriate and thoughtful questions that underlie your interest in the program. Do some research on the medical school before going to the interview. If possible, find out some professional details about the interviewer beforehand. Show that you took the initiative before the interview and are interested in your admission to this program. Examples of questions include:

- What opportunities are there for students to participate in research?
- What opportunities are there for students to participate in community programs?
- Are there opportunities for early-admission students to gain clinical exposure while in college?
- What has your experience been training early-admission students?

Once you are home, it is good form to send a short thank-you letter to each individual with whom you have interviewed. The letter should be addressed appropriately to the interviewer, with proper notation of their status (PhD, MD, etc.). It should be brief, thanking them for having taken the time to interview you. It is helpful to mention how you enjoyed some particular topic discussed during the interview to help them remember who you were. It should also include a quick sentence reaffirming your interest in their program. If you experience any new events, honors, or achievements that may strengthen your application after your interview, send a letter to the program director to describe them and reaffirm your interest in the program.

PART B

PREFACE TO THE PROGRAM PROFILES

The "Program Profiles" section represents the truly unique and invaluable portion of this book. Much of the mystique and lack of awareness of medical school early-admission programs is due to the fact that these programs are not well catalogued and don't share a common title. The annual *AAMC's Medical School Admission Requirements* probably provides the best published account of these programs. However, even their list is limited and incomplete.

We take great pride in providing the most detailed listing of medical school early-admission programs. However, despite researching extensively and cataloguing these programs throughout the country, we must stress that this list is still likely incomplete too. Programs such as those detailed here are constantly evolving. In addition, the parameters, goals, and requirements of these programs change frequently with contract renegotiations between the participating colleges and medical schools.

UNDERSTANDING THE PROGRAM PROFILES

Program Categorization

The catalog of medical school early-admission programs is listed by the state of the participating undergraduate institution. The participating medical schools are listed second. You may see an undergraduate institution listed more than once. That is because some colleges have more than one program with the same or different medical schools. The same goes for medical schools; you may notice medical schools listed multiple times with different undergraduate institutions.

Contact Information

Contact information for both institutions participating in the medical school early-admission program has been provided when applicable. These addresses, phone numbers, and e-mail addresses were retrieved from the respective websites or the *AAMC's Medical School Admissions Requirements: 2014–2015*. As a generalization, it will be more efficient to contact the listed undergraduate office for additional program information. Whenever possible, the formal title of the program and its website URL has been provided. Those websites should be your first stop for obtaining more information about a specific program.

Tuition

Unless otherwise noted, tuition values listed represent the 2014–2015 school year. The values are for tuition only, and they do not include other fees and room and board charges. Also noted are out-of-state tuition for nonresidents whenever applicable, unless the program was limited to in-state residents only. Please note, tuitions change regularly.

The numbers listed may not be always accurate, but they should at least provide a general understanding of an institution's cost.

About the Medical School and the Program

Following the contact information, you will find some general information about the medical school as well as on the medical school early-admission program. The program details, listed as "About the Program," provide as much succinct information possible regarding the goal, organization, and requirements of the medical school early-admission program. Because every program has some particular motivation, we tried to provide the most defining characteristics of each program.

Program Features/Requirements Table

In the table on the bottom of each program profile page, you will find the program's specific title, length, high school requirements, and application deadline. This quick reference section is designed to provide a quick-reference section for each program.

PROGRAM PROFILES

Undergraduate Institution: University of South Alabama
Medical School: University of South Alabama College of Medicine

Undergraduate Contact Information:	Medical School Contact Information:
Office of Admissions	USA College of Medicine,
2500 Meisler Hall	Office of Admissions
390 Alumni Circle	5795 USA Drive N
Mobile, AL 36688-00002	Room 241
(251) 460-6141	Mobile, AL 36688
	(251) 460-7176
2014–2015 tuition: $8,310 ($16, 620 for nonresidents)	*2014–2015 tuition*: $25,471 ($50,492 for nonresidents)
http: //www.southalabama.edu/departments/ admissions/comearlyacceptance.html	

About the Medical School

The College of Medicine at the University of South Alabama is a public institution founded in 1973. The average class size is sixty-five students.

About the Program

Students in their senior year of high school or recent graduates who have not yet entered college are eligible. The program is open to residents of Alabama only. Students accepted into the program must maintain a minimum GPA of 3.5 and a minimum GPA of 3.4 in the sciences and mathematics. The curriculum will consist of core requirements of the selected baccalaureate program and the prerequisites of matriculation to medical school. The MCAT is required, and students must score above the national average. An interview will be conducted with the students after the completion of ninety-six quarter hours to assess the student's academic performance and continued commitment to medicine.

Program Title	The Combined BS/MD Early-admissions Program
Length of Program	8 years
Number of Students	15
High School Requirements	Alabama resident Minimum GPA of 3.5 (unweighted) Minimum SAT score of 1220 (combined critical reading and math) or ACT score of 27
Application Deadline	January 15
MCAT Requirements	Yes (29 or greater)

Undergraduate Institution: University of California, Riverside
Medical School: University of California, Los Angeles School of Medicine

Undergraduate Contact Information: Student Affairs Officer Division of Biomedical Sciences University of California, Riverside Riverside, CA 92521 (908) 787-4333 bmscil@ucracl.ucr.edu	Medical School Contact Information: Office of Admissions UCLA School of Medicine Box 957035 Los Angeles, CA 90095 (310) 825-6081
2014–2015 tuition: $14,800 ($37,678 for nonresidents)	2014–2014 tuition: $35,557 ($47,802 for nonresidents)
http: //medschool.ucr.edu/admissions/haider_program.html	

About the Medical School

The University of California, Los Angeles School of Medicine is a public institution situated on the main UCLA campus. It graduated its first medical school class in 1955. The average class size is 145 students.

About the Program

The Thomas Haider Program in Biomedical Sciences provides an accelerated track to obtaining both the BS and MD degrees in seven years. Students in the program major in biomedical sciences, thus providing extensive background in chemistry, physics, biology, and mathematics, plus exposure to the humanities and social sciences.

In the first three years of the program, students must meet all the requirements of the College of Natural and Agricultural Sciences for a BS degree. Continuation in the program for each student for each of the years is decided by a faculty committee review of academic performance in combination with personal evaluations of each student based on consistent faculty-student contact.

Students are required to take the MCAT during the third year. At the end of the third year at UC-Riverside, selection will be made to identify those individuals who will continue to the medical school phase of the program. Those continuing on to medical school will begin the traditional preclinical medical education at the UC-Riverside campus. The last two years, which comprise the clinical medical education, will be completed at the UCLA School of Medicine.

Program Title	Thomas Haider Program in Biomedical Sciences
Length of Program	7 years (three undergraduate years)
Number of Students	24
High School Requirements	SAT/ACT, SAT II, GPA/Rank required Demonstration of maturity and commitment to medicine

Application Deadline	November 3
MCAT Requirements	Yes (minimum scores not defined)

Undergraduate Institution: University of California, San Diego
Medical School: University of California, San Diego School of Medicine

Undergraduate Contact Information: UC, San Diego 9500 Gilman Dr. La Jolla 92093 (858) 534-2230	*Medical School Contact Information:* Director of Admissions UC, San Diego School of Medicine Office of Admissions 0621 9500 Gilman Drive La Jolla, California 92093 (858) 534-3880
2014–2015 tuition: $13,456 ($22,878 for nonresidents)	*2014–2015 tuition*: $31,134 ($43,379 for nonresidents)
https: //meded.ucsd.edu/groups/med-scholars/overview.html	

About the Medical School

The School of Medicine is a public institution situated on the main campus of UC-San Diego. It has an average class size of 120 students.

About the Program

The Medical Scholars Program has been established to encourage the recruitment of unusually talented high school students to promote the goal of increasing diversity at both of the University of California San Diego undergraduate and medical school campuses.

Program Title	The Medical Scholars Program
Length of Program	8 years
Number of Students	12

High School *Requirements*	Minimum GPA and science GPA of 3.5 (unweighted) Minimum SAT score of 2250 or ACT score of 34
Application Deadline	March 24
MCAT Requirements	None

Undergraduate Institution: University of Connecticut
Medical School: University of Connecticut School of Medicine

Undergraduate Contact Information: University of Connecticut Office of Undergraduate Admissions 2131 Hillside Road, Unit-3088 Storrs, CT 06269-3088 (860) 486-3137	*Medical School Contact Information*: UConn School of Medicine 263 Farmington Avenue Farmington, CT 06030-1905 Phone: (860) 679-2000
2014–2015 tuition: $8,712 ($26,544 for nonresidents)	*2014–2015 tuition*: $34,405 ($63,259 for nonresidents)
http: //admissions.uconn.edu/content/special-program-medicine	

About the Medical School

The University of Connecticut School of Medicine is a public institution established in 1961. The average class size is ninety-eight students. Medical students, in the first week, are assigned to a community physician mentor as they begin their clinical education.

About the Program

This program offers gifted and talented high school students who are focused on a career in medicine the opportunity to combine a broad-based liberal arts program with their medical education. The purpose of this program is to give students more flexibility and diversity in their undergraduate studies.

Program Title	Special Program in Medicine
Length of Program	8 years
High School Requirements	Preference is given to Connecticut residents Minimum SAT score of 1300 (math and critical reading) or ACT score of 29 Minimum GPA of 3.5 (unweighted)
Application Deadline	January 1
MCAT Requirements	Yes (30 or more—with at least 8 on any one section)

Undergraduate Institution: University of Colorado Denver
Medical School: University of Colorado Anschutz Medical Campus

Undergraduate Contact Information:	*Medical School Contact Information*:
University of Colorado Denver BA/BS—MD Program 13120 East 19th Avenue, Room 5229 Aurora, Colorado 80045 (303) 352-3557	Office of Undergraduate Admissions University of Colorado Anschutz Medical Campus Education Tower, II North, Fifth Floor Aurora, Colorado (303) 724-8025 somadmin@ucdenver.edu
2012–2013 tuition: $5,106 ($13,816 for nonresidents)	*2014–2015 tuition*: $34,639 ($60,594 for nonresidents)
http: //www.ucdenver.edu/academics/colleges/CLAS/ BachelorsPrograms/ProgramsDegrees/BABSMD/Pages/home.aspx	

About the Medical School

The University of Colorado Anschutz Medical Campus is a public institution established in 1883. The school of medicine dedicates itself to discovery, innovation, diversity, and the health of the community.

About the Program

This program is designed for students interested especially in the primary care field. This program gives preference to Colorado students. The program encourages the students to stay as physicians in Colorado after training. During their time in college, students are required to attend monthly seminars at Anschutz Medical Campus and participate in summer programs each undergraduate year.

Student just also maintain a cumulative GPA of 3.5 and a science GPA of 3.0 Students must also take the MCAT, but the minimum score is not defined.

Program Title	BA/BS—MD Program
Length of Program	8 years
Number of Students	10
High School Requirements	Preference is given to Colorado residents Minimum CCHE index score of 110 (a combination of GPA or rank, and ACT or SAT score) Minimum GPA of 3.5 (weighted or unweighted) Interest in being a primary care physician.
Application Deadline	October 1
MCAT Requirements	Yes (minimum score not defined)

Undergraduate Institution: George Washington University
Medical School: George Washington University School of Medicine

Undergraduate Contact Information:	*Medical School Contact Information:*
Office of Admissions The George Washington University 2121 I Street, N.W., Suite 201 Washington, DC 20052 (202) 994-6040	Office of Admissions George Washington University School of Medicine Ross Hall, Room 716 2300 Eye Street, NW Washington, DC 20037 (202) 994-3506
2011–2012 tuition: $48,700	*2014–2015 tuition*: $54,183
http: //smhs.gwumc.edu/mdprograms/jointprograms	

About the Medical School

The George Washington School of Medicine is a private institution that opened in 1824. The school of medicine is situated near the main George Washington campus in downtown Washington, DC. The average class size is 150 students.

About the Program

The seven-year BA/MD Program was initiated to provide premedical students the opportunity to explore other fields of interest. The course requirements for the baccalaureate degree in the humanities and social sciences vary, but students must complete thirty-two semester hours in the natural and physical sciences. Accepted students are required to take the MCAT, but it will not be used as a factor for promotion. Students will receive their baccalaureate degrees after completion of the first year of medical school.

Program Title	The 7-Year BA/MD Program
Length of Program	7 years (3 undergraduate years)
Number of Students	10
High School Requirements	Minimum SAT scores of 1400 (combined critical reading and math) or ACT score of 32 SAT II required in math and a science Minimum GPA of at least 3.7 (unweighted) High School rank within the top 5 percent
Application Deadline	December 1
MCAT Requirements	Not required

Undergraduate Institution: St. Bonaventure University
Medical School: George Washington University School of Medicine

Undergraduate Contact Information: Office of Admissions PO Box D St. Bonaventure, NY 14778 (716) 375-2434	*Medical School Contact Information:* Office of Admissions, Room 716 George Washington University School of Medicine 2300 Eye Street, NW Washington, DC 20037 (202) 994-3506
2013–2014 tuition: $29,589	*2014–2015 tuition: $54,183*
http: //www.sbu.edu/academics/schools/arts-and-sciences/departments-majors-minors/premedicine/sbu-gw-dual-admit-program-in-medicine-(m-d-)	

About the Medical School

The George Washington School of Medicine is a private institution that opened in 1825. The School of Medicine is situated near the main George Washington campus in downtown Washington, DC. The average class size is 150 students.

About the Program

This program is for highly qualified high school students who want to maintain both clinical exposure and service work throughout their educational careers. This program is an unaccelerated and unabridged eight-year course with accepted students spending the first four years in the St. Bonaventure University and the next four years in the George Washington School of Medicine and Health Sciences.

Program Title	SBU-GW Dual Admit Program in Medicine
Length of Program	8 years
Number of Students	10 to 15 students
High School Requirements	Minimum SAT scores of 1300 (critical reading and math) or ACT score of 29 SAT II required in a science is preferred
Application Deadline	December 1
MCAT Requirements	Not required

Undergraduate Institution: Howard University
Medical School: Howard University College of Medicine

Undergraduate Contact Information: Office of Admissions Howard University 2400 6th Street, NW Washington, DC 20059	*Medical School Contact Information*: Office of Admissions Howard University College of Medicine 520 W Street, NW Washington, DC 20059 (202) 806-6279
2014–2015 tuition: $12,086	*2012–2013 tuition*: $37,810
http: //healthsciences.howard.edu/education/colleges/ medicine/education/programs-overview/dual-degree	

About the Medical School

The Howard University College of Medicine is a private institution and is the oldest and largest historically black medical school in the country. It opened in 1868. The college's goal is to train students to become competent, compassionate physicians who will provide care in medically underserved communities. There is special attention placed in areas of health care disparities. The average class size is 110 students.

About the Program

The goal of this accelerated combined-degree program is to encourage talented undergraduate students to choose medicine as a career and to retain these students at the Howard University College of Medicine. The program leads to a bachelor's degree awarded by the College of Arts and Sciences and the MD degree by the College of Medicine. Students must complete forty semester hours of humanities and social sciences and at least forty-six semester hours of natural and physical sciences within two years. The MCAT is also required and is to be taken in the spring of the second year. Progression to the medical school is contingent upon the results of the MCAT and GPA.

Program Title	6-Year Combined Degree Program
Length of Program	6 years (two undergraduate years)
Number of Students	10
High School Requirements	Minimum GPA of 3.5 (unweighted) Minimum science GPA of 3.25 Minimum SAT Score of 1950 or ACT of 26
Application Deadline	March 1
MCAT Requirements	Yes (minimum score of 24)

Undergraduate Institution: University of Miami
Medical School: University of Miami School of Medicine

Undergraduate Contact Information: Office of Admission University of Miami PO Box 248025 Coral Gables, Florida 33124-4616 Phone: (305) 284-2211	*Medical School Contact Information*: Office of Admissions University of Miami Miller School of Medicine PO Box 016159 Miami, FL 33101 (305) 243-3234
2014–2014 tuition: $39,980 ($39,980 for nonresidents)	*2011–2012 tuition*: $33,017 ($42,499 for nonresidents)
http: //www.miami.edu/medical-admissions	

About the Medical School

The University of Miami School of Medicine is a private institution and is the largest and oldest medical school in Florida. It was founded in 1952. The School of Medicine is located on the medical campus next to Jackson Memorial Hospital in the Civic Center area of Miami. The average class size is 150 students.

About the Program

The Honors Program in Medicine is the University of Miami's seven- or eight-year BS/MD program. It was established in 1981 and is operated by the School of Medicine in conjunction with the School of Arts and Sciences. It offers exceptionally motivated and talented students who have reached a mature decision to study medicine based on their experiences an opportunity to earn the BS and MD degrees in either seven or eight years.

The first three or four years are spent on the Coral Gables campus of the University of Miami, taking the required courses for their major.

Students must maintain a minimum cumulative GPA of 3.4 and a minimum science GPA of 3.2. Students must also take the MCAT before starting medical school. The MCAT score is not required for promotion but to assess the student's level of preparedness. The baccalaureate degree is received following the first year of medical studies.

Program Title	The Honors Program in Medicine
Length of Program	7 or 8 years (three or four undergraduate years)
Number of Students	20
High School Requirements	GPA of 3.75 SAT score of 1400 (combined math and critical reading) or ACT score of 32 SAT II Subject Tests: 600 minimum in math and one science
Application Deadline	November 1
MCAT Requirements	Yes

Undergraduate Institution: University of Hawaii Manoa
Medical School: University of Hawaii John A. Burns School of Medicine

Undergraduate Contact Information:	Medical School Contact Information:
University of Hawaii at Manoa Office of Admissions 2600 Campus Road, Room 001 Honolulu, HI 96822 (808) 956-8975 uhmanoa.admissions@hawaii.edu	John A. Burns School of Medicine Office of Admissions 651 Ilalo Street, MEB 3rd Floor Honolulu, HI 96813 (808) 692-0892
2014–2015 tuition: $4,920 ($14,316 for nonresidents)	2014–2015 tuition: $16,608 ($33,600 for nonresidents)
http: //manoa.hawaii.edu/admissions/undergrad/early_admissions/	

About the Medical School

The University of Hawaii John A. Burns School of Medicine is a public institution and is the only medical school in Hawaii. It was founded in 1956. The School of Medicine practices "problem-based learning" curriculum to help students learn in a more hands-on approach. The average class size is sixty-six students.

About the Program

Admission to the Doctor of Medicine Early Assurance Program has many benefits to students, including a full tuition scholarship for all four undergraduate years and participation in the honors program. Students in the program work closely with faculty at the school of medicine to already create a relationship before matriculation to the school of medicine. The program only accepts residents of the state Hawaii. Students must also shadow a physician for one semester and gain experience in a nonphysician health career for one semester.

To be promoted, students must maintain a cumulative GPA of 3.5 and a science GPA of 3.4. Students also must get a MCAT score of 30, with no subset below 9, or a MCAT score of 31, with no subset below 8.

Program Title	The Doctor of Medicine Early Assurance Program
Length of Program	7 years (three undergraduate years)
Number of Students	10
High School Requirements	Hawaii resident Minimum GPA of 3.8 (unweighted) Minimum SAT score of 1800 or ACT score of 27
Application Deadline	December 1
MCAT Requirements	Yes (must get achieve a score of 30—with no subset below 9 or achieve a score of 31—with no subset below 8)

Undergraduate Institution: Northwestern University
Medical School: Northwestern University Medical School

Undergraduate Contact Information:	Medical School Contact Information:
Office of Admission and Financial Aid PO Box 3060 1801 Hinman Avenue Evanston, IL 60204 (708) 491-7271 ug-admissions@nwu.edu	Honors Program in Medical Education 303 E. Chicago Avenue Ward Building 1-003 Chicago, IL 60611-3008 (312) 503-8915 hpme@northwestern.edu
2014–2015 tuition: $43,380	*2014–2015 tuition*: $51,882
http: //www.feinberg.northwestern.edu/education/ degree-programs/hpme/index.html	

About the Medical School

Northwestern University Medical School is a private institution founded in 1859. The medical campus is situated at Northwestern University's lakefront Chicago campus. The medical students gain clinical experience at the McGaw Hospitals, which is a group of urban, suburban, specialized, and general hospitals throughout the Chicago area. The average class size is 165 students.

About the Program

Northwestern's Honors Program in Medical Education is an accelerated program that can be completed in seven years or the standard eight years. The first three or four years of the program are spent on the Evanston campus, and the last four are spent at the medical school on the lakefront Chicago campus. Students may choose one of several options to complete their undergraduate career, culminating in a BA or BS degree, prior to proceeding to medical school. In the Weinberg College of Arts and Sciences, the student may pursue an honors-level concentration in a specific department. The School of Speech offers students an opportunity to study communication sciences. Also, students may major in biomedical engineering in the McCormick School of Engineering and Applied Science. Students may take time off between undergraduate studies and matriculation to medical school to pursue research, other degrees, international opportunities, and other areas of personal interest. This program is designed to be customizable to the students' career goals.

Program Title	The BA/MD Honors Program in Medical Education
Length of Program	7–8 years (3–4 undergraduate years)
Number of Students	40
High School Requirements	The SAT or ACT required The SAT II (in mathematics IIC, chemistry, writing) required
Application Deadline	January 1
MCAT Requirements	None

Undergraduate Institution: Indiana State University
Medical School: Indiana University School of Medicine

Undergraduate Contact Information:	*Medical School Contact Information*:
Office of Admissions Indiana State University John W. Moore Welcome Center 318 North Sixth Street Terre Haute, IN 47809 (812) 237-2121	IUSM Office of Admissions Fesler Hall 213 1120 South Drive Indianapolis, IN 46202 (317) 274-3772 inmedadm@iupui.edu
2014–2015 tuition: $8,216 ($18,146 for nonresidents)	*2014–2015 tuition*: $32,691 ($50,132 for nonresidents)
http: //www.indstate.edu/preprof/rhp.htm	

About the Medical School

The Indiana University School of Medicine is a public institution founded in 1903. It is the only medical school in the state. The school has multiple campuses throughout Indiana where students can spend the first two years of medical school. The average class size is 280 students.

About the Program

The BA/MD Rural Health Program is designed to address the rural health needs of the state of Indiana by providing increased opportunities for residents from rural communities to obtain education and training in medicine. During the undergraduate component of the program, students enrolled in the rural health program will participate in special experiences designed to enhance their careers as medical practitioners in rural settings. The curriculum will be a traditional premed curriculum that has been modified to enhance the likelihood of success in the practice of rural medicine.

Admissions into the program will be limited to Indiana residents from rural communities. Accepted students are required to maintain a minimum cumulative GPA of 3.5 and take the MCAT for promotion to the medical school.

Program Title	BA/MD Rural Health Program
Length of Program	8 years
Number of Students	10
High School Requirements	Indiana resident SAT score of 1200 (combined critical reading and math) or ACT score of 27 GPA of 3.5
Application Deadline	December 1
MCAT Requirements	Yes (must achieve a score equal to the mean of the previous year's matriculating class)

Undergraduate Institution: University of Kentucky
Medical School: University of Kentucky College of Medicine

Undergraduate Contact Information: Assistant Director of Admission for Recruitment University of Kentucky 12 W. D. Funkhouser Building Lexington, KY 40506 Phone: (859) 218-1360	Medical School Contact Information: College of Medicine Office of Medical Education 138 Leader Ave. Rm. 109 Lexington, KY 40506-9983
2014–2015 tuition: $10,616 ($22,888 for nonresidents)	2014–2015 tuition: $33,899 ($60,545 for nonresidents)
http: //meded.med.uky.edu/bs-md-program-overview	

About the Medical School

The University of Kentucky College of Medicine is a private institution founded in 1960. The College of Medicine is located in Lexington, Kentucky. The average class size is 136 students.

About the Program

This program gives gifted and talented high school students who are certain that they want to become physicians or physician-scientists the opportunity to combine and accelerate their undergraduate and professional education at the University of Kentucky. This program gives students a chance to shadow other physicians while in the program. The program also provides several enrichment programs designed to help the students get acquainted with research, clinical, and community service experiences.

Accepted students are required to maintain a minimum cumulative GPA of 3.5 and take the MCAT for promotion to the medical school.

Program Title	BS/MD Program
Length of Program	7 years (three undergraduate years)
Number of Students	5 to 10
High School Requirements	Minimum SAT score of 1360 (combined critical reading and math) or ACT score of 31 Minimum GPA of 3.5 (unweighted)
Application Deadline	November 15
MCAT Requirements	Yes (minimum score is not defined)

Undergraduate Institution: Boston University
Medical School: Boston University School of Medicine

Undergraduate Contact Information: Boston University Admissions 881 Commonwealth Avenue 6th floor, Admissions Boston, MA 02215 (617) 353-2300 admissions@bu.edu	Medical School Contact Information: Admissions Office Boston University School of Medicine 72 E. Concord St. L-124 Boston, MA 02118 (617) 638-4630 medadms@bu.edu
2014–2015 tuition: $45,686	2014–2015 tuition: $51,548
http: //www.bu.edu/academics/cas/programs/ seven-year-liberal-arts-medical-education-program/	

About the Medical School

The Boston University School of Medicine is a private institution founded in 1873 by Boston University at the site of the original New England Female Medical College. The School of Medicine is part of the larger Boston Medical Center. The average class size is 150 students.

About the Program

The Seven-Year Liberal Arts / Medical Education Program integrates the undergraduate and medical school curriculum, thereby shortening the overall period of study. Students who are accepted into the program are admitted to the College of Arts and Sciences and provisionally to Boston University School of Medicine. The combined curriculum offers extensive elective options for study in the humanities and social sciences. The flexible nature of the program allows students to develop their academic interests while fulfilling premedical requirements at an accelerated and more rigorous level. Students receive their bachelor of arts degree in medical science at the completion of the fourth year (which constitutes their first full year of medical study as graduate students) and the doctor of medicine degree at the completion of the seventh year. Students may also choose an eight-year version of the program—where the students in good academic standing continue their fourth academic year.

Program Title	The Seven-Year Liberal Arts / Medical Education Program
Length of Program	7 years (three undergraduate years)
Number of Students	20
High School Requirements	The SAT or ACT, and class rank required. The SAT II (mathematics II, and chemistry) (required) SAT II in foreign language (recommended) Minimum GPA of 3.9
Application Deadline	December 1
MCAT Requirements	Yes (minimum score of 30)

Undergraduate Institution: University of Missouri, Kansas City
Medical School: University of Missouri, Kansas City School of Medicine

Undergraduate Contact Information: UMKC Office of Admissions 120 Administrative Center University of Missouri- Kansas City 5100 Rockhill Road Kansas City, MO 64110-2499 (816) 235–1111	Medical School Contact Information: Council on Selection UMKC School of Medicine 2411 Holmes Kansas City, MO 64108 (816) 235–1870 or 1783
2013–2014 tuition: $9,456 ($22,203 for nonresidents)	2014–2015 tuition: $28,719 ($57,438 for nonresidents)
http: //www.umkc.edu/degrees/Md.asp	

About the Medical School

The University of Missouri, Kansas City School of Medicine is a public institution founded in 1969. Located on suburban Hospital Hill campus, the medical school is near both the schools and colleges of the university and affiliated hospitals. The average class size is one hundred students.

About the Program

The University of Missouri, Kansas City School of Medicine's primary educational mission is a combined baccalaureate / doctor of medicine degree program directly out of high school. It is an integrated program with a mix of liberal arts, basic medical sciences, and clinical medicine throughout the curriculum. The program has ongoing clinical involvement that begins from the first year and progressively increases. The program features an eleven-month curriculum with a one-month vacation and structures academic and clinical experiences to provide both degrees in six years from the same institution. Students spend three-quarters of their time the first two years working toward their baccalaureate requirements. Conversely, students spend three-quarters of their last four years completing their MD requirements. Thereby, the study of medicine and liberal arts are integrated for all six years.

Program Title	The School of Medicine Six-Year Program
Length of Program	6 years
Number of Students	120
High School Requirements	Missouri residents: top 20 percent of class and ACT minimum of 26 Non-Missouri residents: top 10 percent of class and ACT minimum of 28 or SAT composite of 1200 (critical reading and math)
Application Deadline	November 1
MCAT Requirements	None

Undergraduate Institution: Caldwell University
Medical School: Rutgers—New Jersey Medical School

Undergraduate Contact Information:	Medical School Contact Information:
Health Professions Adviser 120 Bloomfield Avenue Caldwell, NJ 07006 Phone: (973) 618-3595 vukachukwu@caldwell.edu	New Jersey Medical School Office of Admissions Medical Sciences Building Room C-653 185 South Orange Avenue Newark, NJ 07103 (973) 972-4631 njmsadmiss@njms.rutgers.edu
2014–2015 tuition: $28,900	2014–2015 tuition: $35,823 ($57,479 for nonresidents)
http://www.caldwell.edu/academics/ health-professions/health-professions-faqs#ap1	

About the Medical School

The New Jersey Medical School of Rutgers University is a public institution established in Newark, New Jersey, in 1977. The average medical school class size is 170 students. The New Jersey Medical School has established accelerated baccalaureate/MD-degree programs in collaboration with different undergraduate institutions. The goal of these programs is to give highly qualified high school students an opportunity to broaden their premedical preparation without having to compete for admission to medical school.

About the Program

This program was created to give the students an opportunity to obtain a liberal arts degree along with preparing them for medical school. Students must maintain a cumulative and science GPA of 3.5, getting no grade less than a B in all science classes. Also, students must engage in research at the New Jersey Medical School over a summer during their undergraduate studies. Finally, although no minimum score is required on the test, students must also sit for the MCAT.

Program Title	7-year BA/MD Rutgers-New Jersey Medical School Affiliation Program
Length of Program	7 years (3 undergraduate years)
Number of Students	5 to 10 students
High School Requirements	Minimum SAT score of 1400 (combined critical reading and math) Minimum high school rank in the top 10 percent
Application Deadline	December 1
MCAT Requirements	Yes (no minimum requirement)

Undergraduate Institution: The College of New Jersey
Medical School: Rutgers—New Jersey Medical School

Undergraduate Contact Information:	Medical School Contact Information:
Chairman, Medical Careers Committee The College of New Jersey PO Box 7718 Ewing, NJ 08628-0718 Phone: (609) 771-2021 morrisja@tcnj.edu	New Jersey Medical School Office of Admissions Medical Sciences Building Room C-653 185 South Orange Avenue Newark, NJ 07103 (973) 972-4631 njmsadmiss@njms.rutgers.edu
2013–2014 tuition: $14,730 ($25,135 for nonresidents)	*2014–2015 tuition*: $35,823 ($57,479 for nonresidents)
http: //biology.pages.tcnj.edu/academics/ medical-careers/seven-year-medical-program/	

About the Medical School

The New Jersey Medical School of Rutgers University is a public institution established in Newark, New Jersey, in 1977. The average medical school class size is 170 students. The New Jersey Medical School has established accelerated baccalaureate/MD-degree programs in collaboration with different undergraduate institutions. The goal of these programs is to give highly qualified high school students an opportunity to broaden their premedical preparation without having to compete for admission to medical school.

About the Program

As a participant in the program, students must maintain an overall minimum GPA of 3.5/4.0, and earn a B or better in each basic required medical school course. Also, students must engage in research at the New Jersey Medical School over a summer during their undergraduate studies. Finally, although no minimum score is required on the test, students must also sit for the MCAT. However, it is recommended to achieve the national mean score of 31.

Program Title	The 7-Year Combined BS/MD Program
Length of Program	7 years (3 undergraduate years)
Number of Students	20 students
High School Requirements	Minimum SAT Score of 1480 (combined critical reading and math on one test date) Minimum GPA of 4.5 or 95 percent Must be in the top 5 percent of high school class
Application Deadline	December 1
MCAT Requirements	Yes (no minimum but recommended achieving a score of 31)

Undergraduate Institution: Drew University
Medical School: Rutgers,—New Jersey Medical School

Undergraduate Contact Information: College Admissions Drew University Madison, NJ Phone: (973) 408-3739 cadm@drew.edu	Medical School Contact Information: New Jersey Medical School Office of Admissions Medical Sciences Building Room C-653 185 South Orange Avenue Newark, NJ 07103 (973) 972-4631 njmsadmiss@njms.rutgers.edu
2014–2015 tuition: $41,688	2014–2015 tuition: $35,823 ($57,479 for nonresidents)
http: //www.drew.edu/undergraduate/ what-you-learn/premed/dual-degree	

About the Medical School

The New Jersey Medical School of Rutgers University is a public institution established in Newark, New Jersey, in 1977. The average medical school class size is 170 students. The New Jersey Medical School has established accelerated baccalaureate/MD-degree programs in collaboration with different undergraduate institutions. The goal of these programs is to give highly qualified high school students an opportunity to broaden their premedical preparation without having to compete for admission to medical school.

About the Program

The College of Liberal Arts of Drew University sponsors this program where students in the program may major in any liberal arts concentration. The required premedical courses must be completed within the three-year period at Drew, in addition to the requirements of the selected major and the general education requirements for the liberal arts degree.

Students must maintain an overall minimum GPA of 3.4 each semester. In addition, students must maintain a minimum science GPA of 3.4 each semester at Drew, with a minimum of B- in each of the required premedical courses. Finally, although no minimum score is required on the test for candidates who have remained in good academic standing, students must also sit for the MCAT during their junior year.

Program Title	The Dual Degree Medical Program
Length of Program	7 years
Number of Students	5 to 10 students
High School Requirements	Minimum SAT score of 1500 (combined critical reading and math) or ACT of 34 Minimum GPA of 3.8 (unweighted) High school rank in the top 10 percent (minimum required)

Application Deadline	December 1
MCAT Requirements	Yes (no minimum requirement)

Undergraduate Institution: Montclair State University
Medical School: Rutgers—New Jersey Medical School

Undergraduate Contact Information:	*Medical School Contact Information:*
Montclair State University	Office of Admissions
Undergraduate Admissions	Medical Sciences Building
College Hall, Room 100	Room C-653
One Normal Avenue	185 South Orange Avenue
Montclair, NJ 07043	Newark, NJ 07103
(973) 655-3418	(973) 972-4631
HazardL@mail.montclair.edu	njmsadmiss@njms.rutgers.edu
2014–2015 tuition: $11,318 ($20,196 for nonresidents)	*2014–2015 tuition*: $35,823 ($57,479 for nonresidents)
https: //www.montclair.edu/csam/health-careers/combined-bs-md/	

About the Medical School

The New Jersey Medical School of Rutgers University is a public institution established in Newark, New Jersey, in 1977. The average medical school class size is 170 students. The New Jersey Medical School has established accelerated baccalaureate/MD-degree programs in collaboration with different undergraduate institutions. The goal of these programs is to give highly qualified high school students an opportunity to broaden their premedical preparation without having to compete for admission to medical school.

About the Program

As participants in this program, students will join the MSU Honors Program. The students will also be provided summer and academic-year enrichment activities. To advance to the medical school, students must achieve a minimum grade of a B in all science courses. Students must also maintain a cumulative and semester GPA of at least 3.2. Although the MCAT is required, there is no minimum required score.

Program Title	The Health Careers Combined BS/MD Program
Length of Program	8 years
Number of Students	No quota
High School Requirements	Highly motivated and academically capable from financially and educationally disadvantaged backgrounds Minimum SAT score of 1100 (combined critical reading and math in one test sitting—with no subset less than 550) Minimum high school rank in the top 10 percent Minimum cumulative and science GPA of a B
Application Deadline	December 15
MCAT Requirements	Yes (no minimum required score)

Undergraduate Institution: New Jersey Institute of Technology
Medical School: Rutgers—New Jersey Medical School

Undergraduate Contact Information:	Medical School Contact Information:
Albert Dorman Honors College New Jersey Institute of Technology 323 Martin Luther King Jr. Blvd. Newark, NJ 07102 Phone: (973) 642-7664, (973) 596-5442 dhawan@adm.njit.edu	Office of Admissions Medical Sciences Building Room C-653 185 South Orange Avenue Newark, NJ 07103 (973) 972-4631 njmsadmiss@njms.rutgers.edu

2014–2015 tuition: $12,800 ($25,856 for nonresidents)	*2014–2015 tuition*: $35,823 ($57,479 for nonresidents)
http: //honors.njit.edu/	

About the Medical School

The New Jersey Medical School of Rutgers University is a public institution established in Newark, New Jersey, in 1977. The average medical school class size is 170 students. The New Jersey Medical School has established accelerated baccalaureate/MD-degree programs in collaboration with different undergraduate institutions. The goal of these programs is to give highly qualified high school students an opportunity to broaden their premedical preparation without having to compete for admission to medical school.

About the Program

The BS/MD Program is an accelerated seven-year program. In the program, students study for three years at NJIT, followed by the traditional four years of medical school. Students are awarded a bachelors degree in engineering science upon the successful completion of their first year of professional studies at the New Jersey Medical School. As a participant in the program, students must maintain an overall minimum GPA of 3.4 and maintain a minimum science GPA of 3.4. Also, students must engage in research at the New Jersey Medical School over a summer during their undergraduate studies. Finally, although no minimum score is required on the test, students must also sit for the MCAT. Students accepted into this program will also receive a scholarship that covers their full cost of attendance.

Program Title	The 7-Year Accelerated BS/MD Program
Length of Program	7 years (3 undergraduate years)
Number of Students	No quota

High School Requirements	Minimum SAT score of 1400 (combined critical reading and math on one test) or ACT score of 32 High school rank in the top 10 percent
Application Deadline	December 1
MCAT Requirements	Yes (no minimum required score)

Undergraduate Institution: Rutgers University—Newark Campus
Medical School: Rutgers—New Jersey Medical School

Undergraduate Contact Information: Office of Admissions 312 Hill Hall 360 Dr. MLK Jr. Blvd. Newark, NJ 07012-1801 (973) 353-5800 sopinto@rutgers.edu	Medical School Contact Information: Office of Admissions Medical Sciences Building Room C-653 185 South Orange Avenue Newark, NJ 07103 (973) 972-4631 njmsadmiss@njms.rutgers.edu
2014–2015 tuition: $13,499 ($27,523 for nonresidents)	2014–2015 tuition: $35,823 ($57,479 for nonresidents)
http: //www.ncas.rutgers.edu/oas/bamd-program-nwk-applying	

About the Medical School

The New Jersey Medical School of Rutgers University is a public institution established in Newark, New Jersey, in 1977. The average medical school class size is 170 students. The New Jersey Medical School has established accelerated baccalaureate/MD-degree programs in collaboration with different undergraduate institutions. The goal of these programs is to give highly qualified high school students an opportunity to broaden their premedical preparation without having to compete for admission to medical school.

About the Program

The purpose of this joint articulated program is to permit integration of basic medical sciences into advanced natural science courses in preparing students for the clinical portion of their professional educations. Students accepted into this program must maintain an overall minimum GPA of 3.4 and a minimum science GPA of 3.4. Also, students must engage in research at the New Jersey Medical School over a summer during their undergraduate studies. Finally, although no minimum score is required on the test, students must also sit for the MCAT.

Program Title	Joint Bachelor / Medical Degree Program
Length of Program	7 years (3 undergraduate years)
Number of Students	No quota
High School Requirements	Minimum SAT score of 1400 (combined critical reading and math on one test) or ACT score of 32 High school rank in the top 10 percent
Application Deadline	November 1
MCAT Requirements	Yes—no minimum required score

Undergraduate Institution: Stevens Institute of Technology
Medical School: Rutgers—New Jersey Medical School

Undergraduate Contact Information:	*Medical School Contact Information:*
Office of Undergraduate Admissions	Office of Admissions
1 Castle Point on Hudson	Medical Sciences Building
Howe Center, 8th floor	Room C-653
Hoboken, NJ 07030	185 South Orange Avenue
(201) 216-5194	Newark, NJ 07103
efleming@stevens.edu	(973) 972-4631
	njmsadmiss@njms.rutgers.edu

2014–2015 tuition: $22,105	2014–2015 tuition: $35,823 ($57,479 for nonresidents)
http://www.stevens.edu/sit/admissions/ academics/preprofessional.cfm	

About the Medical School

The New Jersey Medical School of Rutgers University is a public institution established in Newark, New Jersey, in 1977. The average medical school class size is 170 students. The New Jersey Medical School has established accelerated baccalaureate/MD-degree programs in collaboration with different undergraduate institutions. The goal of these programs is to give highly qualified high school students an opportunity to broaden their premedical preparation without having to compete for admission to medical school.

About the Program

This is an accelerated program where three years are initially spent at the Stevens Institute of Technology, followed by the traditional four years of medical school. As a participant in the program, students must maintain an overall minimum GPA of 3.4 and maintain a minimum science GPA of 3.4. Also, students must engage in research at the New Jersey Medical School over a summer during their undergraduate studies. Finally, although no minimum score is required on the test, students must also sit for the MCAT.

Program Title	The 7-Year BS/MD Program
Length of Program	7 years (3 undergraduate years)
Number of Students	No quota

High School Requirements	Minimum SAT score of 1400 (combined critical reading and math in one test sitting) SAT II in Mathematics level I or II, and biology or chemistry Minimum high school rank in the top 10 percent
Application Deadline	January 1
MCAT Requirements	Yes (no minimum required score)

Undergraduate Institution: University of New Mexico
Medical School: University of New Mexico School of Medicine

Undergraduate Contact Information: Office of Admissions University of New Mexico 1155 University Blvd. SE, Albuquerque, NM, 87131 (505) 277-8900	*Medical School Contact Information*: Admissions Committee UNM School of Medicine MSC09 5065 1 University of New Mexico Albuquerque, NM 87131-0001 (505) 925-4500 combinedbamd@salud.unm.edu
2014–2015 tuition: $6,447 ($20,688 for nonresidents)	*2010-2011 tuition*: $16,170 ($46,347 for nonresidents)
http: //som.unm.edu/bamd/index.html	

About the Medical School

The University of New Mexico School of Medicine is a public institution that was founded in 1964. The school of medicine had the main goal of helping alleviate the shortage of doctors in the community. Since then, the University of New Mexico School of Medicine has become a vital part of the community by implementing 141 programs for the surrounding communities.

About the Program

This program is open only to New Mexico residents and was created to help address the shortage of physicians in New Mexico. The students chosen for the program are expected to help serve New Mexico communities. There is no minimum MCAT score requirement. Students must be in good academic standing to matriculate.

Program Title	Combined BA/MD Degree
Length of Program	8 years
Number of Students	28
High School Requirements	Must be a New Mexico resident Minimum SAT math score of 510 and SAT critical reading score of 450, or ACT math score of 22, ACT reading score of 18, ACT science score 19, and ACT English score of 19 Volunteer experience Committed to help serve New Mexico
Application Deadline	November 14
MCAT Requirements	Yes—no minimum required score

Undergraduate Institution: Brooklyn College
Medical School: SUNY—Downstate Medical Center College of Medicine

Undergraduate Contact Information:	*Medical School Contact Information:*
Director, BA/MD Program	Director of Admission
222 West Quad Center	SUNY—Health Science
Brooklyn College	Center at Brooklyn
2900 Bedford Avenue	450 Clarkson Avenue—Box 60M
Brooklyn, NY 11210	Brooklyn, NY 11203
(718) 951-5001	(718) 270-2446
adminqry@brooklyn.cuny.edu	admissions@downstate.edu
2014–2015 tuition: $7,063 ($16,183 for nonresidents)	*2014–2015 tuition*: $35,090 ($60,250 for nonresidents)
http: //www.brooklyn.cuny.edu/web/academics/ honors/academy/programs/ba-md.php	

About the Medical School

The State University of New York (SUNY)—Downstate Medical Center is a public institution founded originally as a part of Long Island College Hospital in 1860. In 1950, the medical school officially joined the SUNY system. The average class size is 180 students.

About the Program

The program aims to produce physicians who are humanists, concerned with the caring as well as curing dimensions of medicine, and to offer an economically affordable baccalaureate and medical school education. Students must maintain a minimum cumulative GPA of 3.5 and a minimum science GPA of 3.5. Students must also take the MCAT during their junior year and score a minimum of 9 on all three sections to be promoted to the medical school.

Program Title	The BA / MD Program
Length of Program	8 years
Number of Students	15
High School Requirements	Preference is given to New York residents Minimum SAT score of 1200 (combined critical reading and math) Average cumulative grade of 90 percent (minimum)
Application Deadline	December 31
MCAT Requirements	Yes (must achieve a minimum score of 9 in all three sections)

Undergraduate Institution: Rensselaer Polytechnic Institute
Medical School: Albany Medical College

Undergraduate Contact Information: Dean of Undergraduate Admissions Rensselaer Polytechnic Institute 110 Eight Street Troy, NY 12180 (518) 276-6216 admissions@rpi.edu	Medical School Contact Information: Office of Admissions, Mail Code 3 Albany Medical College 47 New Scotland Avenue Albany, NY 12208 (518) 262-5521 admissions@mail.amc.edu
2014–2052 tuition: $34,900	2014–2015 tuition: $52,160
http: //admissions.rpi.edu/undergraduate/academics/accelerated.html	

About the Medical School

The Albany Medical College is a private institution founded in 1839. The college buildings and those of the Albany Medical Center Hospital are physically joined in one large complex that comprises the Albany Medical Center. The average class size is 130 students.

About the Program

The Accelerated Physician-Scientist Program offers qualified individuals the opportunity to become physicians who are also intensively trained in medical research. This program looks for students interested in closing the gap between the laboratory and the patient by identifying students who will conduct biomedical research to improve the health of the country as a whole. This approach provides a well-rounded perspective that prepares future practitioners and physician-scientists to perform with confidence and care in a technologically changing environment.

Program Title	The Accelerated Physician-Scientist Program
Length of Program	7 years (3 undergraduate years)
Number of Students	20
High School Requirements	SAT, class rank, and SAT II (in math and a science) required The ACT may be taken in place of the SAT I
Application Deadline	December 1
MCAT Requirements	None

Undergraduate Institution: University of Rochester
Medical School: University of Rochester School of Medicine and Dentistry

Undergraduate Contact Information:	*Medical School Contact Information*:
University of Rochester Office of Admissions PO Box 270251 Rochester, NY 14627 (585) 275-3221 admit@admissions.rochester.edu	University of Rochester School of Medicine and Dentistry Office of Admission 601 Elmwood Avenue, Box 706 Rochester, NY 14642 Room 1–5408 (585) 275-3030

2014–2015 tuition: $46,150	*2014–2015 tuition*: $48,600
http: //enrollment.rochester.edu/admissions/caps/	

About the Medical School

The School of Medicine and Dentistry is a private institution established by the University of Rochester in 1920. The School of Medicine professes the biopsychosocial model of learning that is a student-centered educational program. The average class size is one hundred students. The school has a double-helix curriculum where the school combines clinical work with medical school classes.

About the Program

The Rochester Early Medical Scholars Program is an eight-year program designed for exceptionally talented undergraduates. Students enrolled in this program enter the University of Rochester with an assurance of admission to the university's School of Medicine and Dentistry when they complete their undergraduate degree programs, provided that they maintain a high level of academic achievement, fulfill college and departmental requirements, and complete required premedical courses. The program allows the utmost flexibility in degree programs, mentoring relationships with medical school staff, and early exposure to medical school curriculum through a series of lectures and seminars. The students work closely with respected faculty, gain experience in labs, and get funding for summer research projects.

In the program, students must maintain a minimum cumulative GPA of 3.3 and a minimum premedical courses GPA of 3.3 by the end of sophomore year. Students must have a minimum cumulative GPA of 3.5 by the time of their undergraduate graduation.

Program Title	The Rochester Early Medical Scholars Program
Length of Program	8 years
Number of Students	10–15
High School Requirements	SAT required (students enrolled had average SAT above 1400 combined critical reading and math) Top 3 percent of class (usually have GPA of 3.95)
Application Deadline	December 1
MCAT Requirements	None

Undergraduate Institution: Sophie Davis School of Biomedical Education
Medical School: City University of New York Medical School

Undergraduate Contact Information: Office of Admissions The Sophie Davis School of Biomedical Education Harris Hall 101 160 Convent Avenue New York, NY 10031 (212) 650-7718 sdadmissions@med.cuny.edu	Medical School Contact Information: N / A
2014–2015 tuition: $6,030	2014–2015 tuition: N / A
http: //www.ccny.cuny.edu/sophiedavis/bsmd.cfm	

About the Medical School

The medical school portion of this program involves the final two years of the seven-year program and is completed at one of the following six medical schools where the MD degree will be conferred: Albany Medical College, New York Medical College, New York University

School of Medicine, Northeast Ohio Medical University College of Medicine, SUNY—Brooklyn, or the Commonwealth Medical College.

This program is in response to the continuing shortage of primary care physicians in our nation. Note: All students entering the program must sign a postgraduate service commitment agreement promising to provide primary care medical services in a New York State medically-underserved urban community for a period of two years following their residency training.

About the Program

The Biomedical Education Program is designed as a seven-year integrated curriculum. During the first five years of the program, students fulfill all requirements for the BS degree as well as the preclinical portion of a medical school curriculum. After successfully completing the five-year sequence and passing step 1 of the US Medical Licensure Examination, students transfer to one of the above listed six medical schools for their final two years of clinical training. The BS degree is conferred by City College, while the medical school to which the student transfers awards the MD degree.

Program Title	The BS / MD Program
Length of Program	7 years (3 undergraduate years)
Number of Students	60
High School Requirements	SAT scores or ACT scores required Must be a New York resident
Application Deadline	January 9
MCAT Requirements	None

Undergraduate Institution: State University of New York at Stony Brook
Medical School: SUNY—Stony Brook School of Medicine Health
Science Center

Undergraduate Contact Information:	*Medical School Contact Information*:
Scholars for Medicine Program	Office Of Admissions
The Honors College	Health Sciences Tower,
SUNY at Stony Brook	Level 4—Room 147a
279 Broadway	Stony Brook, New
Albany, NY 12204-2755	York 11794-8434
(631) 632-6868	(631) 444-2113
	somadmissions@
	stonybrookmedicine.edu
2014–2015 tuition: $6,170 ($19,590 for nonresidents)	*2014–2015 tuition*: $35,090 ($60,250 for nonresidents)
http: //www.stonybrook.edu/ugadmissions/ newhonors/scholarsmed.shtml	

About the Medical School

The SUNY—Stony Brook School of Medicine is a public institution,
established in 1971. It is a part of the Stony Brook Health Science
Center, which includes the University Hospital. The average class size
is one hundred students.

About the Program

The Scholars for Medicine Program is a special track within the Honors
College, reserved for a small number of students who intend to pursue
careers in medicine. This eight-year program was designed for high-
achieving students who want a solid liberal arts education before
entering medical school. Accepted students have access to a wide array

of liberal arts courses offered through the university and its Honors College.

A seat in Stony Brook's School for Medicine is reserved for each Scholar for Medicine who successfully completes the four-year Honors College program, maintains a minimum 3.4 GPA, completes all the required premedical courses successfully, and attains a cumulative MCAT score comparable to the national average of medical school matriculates.

Program Title	Scholars for Medicine Program
Length of Program	8 years
Number of Students	5
High School Requirements	Minimum SAT score of 1350 (combined critical reading and math) Minimum GPA of 3.8 (unweighted)
Application Deadline	January 15
MCAT Requirements	Yes (must meet the national average with no score below 8 in any section)

Undergraduate Institution: Union College
Medical School: Albany Medical College

Undergraduate Contact Information:	*Medical School Contact Information*:
Associate Dean of Admissions Union College 807 Union Street Schenectady, NY 12308 (518) 388-6112 admissions@union.edu	Office of Admissions, Mail Code 3 Albany Medical College 47 New Scotland Avenue Albany, NY 12208 (518) 262-5521 admissions@mail.amc.edu
2014–2015 tuition: $48,384	*2014–2015 tuition*: $52,160
http: //www.union.edu/offices/lim/about/	

About the Medical School

The Albany Medical College is a private institution founded in 1839. The college buildings and those of the Albany Medical Center Hospital are physically joined in one large complex that comprises the Albany Medical Center. The average class size is 130 students.

About the Program

The Leadership in Medicine/Health Systems Program is specifically designed for students who want to prepare for the challenge of medical leadership by taking advantage of additional educational opportunities as part of their undergraduate educations. Program students will complete an interdepartmental major in humanities or social sciences and a special program in biomedical ethics that will prepare them for extensive training in medical ethics that they will receive at the Albany Medical College. Students also will complete a term of study abroad where they will be exposed to the health care systems of other countries and a master's-level program in health care management at Union's Graduate Management Institute. Additionally, while they are at Union, students will have the option of also earning a master's in business administration (MBA) with five additional courses.

Program Title	The Leadership in Medicine/Health Systems Program
Length of Program	8 years
Number of Students	15–20
High School Requirements	Minimum SAT score of 2010 or ACT score of 30 Minimum SAT II scores of 650 High school class rank within top 10 percent
Application Deadline	November 15
MCAT Requirements	No requirement

Undergraduate Institution: East Carolina University
Medical School: Brody School of Medicine at East Carolina University

Undergraduate Contact Information: Honors College 101 Mamie Jenkins Building East Carolina University Greenville, NC 27858 (252) 328-6373 honorscollege@ecu.edu	*Medical School Contact Information:* Office of Admissions Brody School of Medicine at East Carolina University 600 Moye Boulevard East Carolina University Greenville, NC 27858 (252) 744-2202 somadmissions@ecu.edu
2014–2015 tuition: $6,143 ($21,340 for nonresidents)	*2014–2052 tuition*: $16,950
http: //www.ecu.edu/cs-acad/earlyassurance/medicine.cfm	

About the Medical School

The Brody School of Medicine at East Carolina University is a public institution started in 1974. The medical school is dedicated to providing excellence in education, research, and clinical services.

About the Program

This program is created for students interested in continuing their educations at Brody School of Medicine. The students must first be accepted into the Honors College at East Carolina University to be considered for admission into the Early Assurance Program. This program also includes hands-on medical exposure, summer programs, and service learning. Students in the program are exempt from taking the MCAT.

Program Title	Early Assurance Program
Length of Program	8 years
Number of Students	4
High School Requirements	Minimum SAT score of 1200 (combined critical reading and math) or ACT score of 27 High school rank/GPA of 3.5 (unweighted) or 4.0 (weighted)
Application Deadline	November 15
MCAT Requirements	None

Undergraduate Institution: University of Akron
Medical School: Northeastern Ohio Medical University

Undergraduate Contact Information:	Medical School Contact Information:
The University of Akron Office of Admissions Simmons Hall 109 Akron, OH 44325-2001 (330) 972-7100	Director of Admissions Northeastern Ohio Medical University 4209 State Route 44, PO Box 95 Rootstown, OH 44272 (330) 325-6270 admission@neomed.edu
2014–2015 tuition: $9,920 ($19,316 for nonresidents)	2014–2052 tuition: $36,950 ($44,915 for nonresidents)
http: //www.neomed.edu/admissions/medicine/bsmd	

About the Medical School

Northeastern Ohio Medical University (NEOMED) is a public institution dedicated to primary care. The medical school maintains its preclinical campus in Rootstown, Ohio. Clinical training occurs at sixteen local community hospitals. The average class size is 130 students, 105 of which are from the three BS/MD programs sponsored by Northeastern Ohio Medical University.

About the Program

The program is designed to allow motivated and bright students the opportunity to complete their premedical and medical education in less time, either six or seven years—with two to three being the undergraduate years—without the stress of medical school admissions. Northeastern Ohio Medical University (NEOMED) offers this program with three undergraduate universities (the University of Akron, Kent State University, and Youngstown State University), which are all within a thirty-five-mile radius of the medical school. The program is open to all students, but preference is given to Ohio residents. Each university has its own BS/MD admissions committee, interviews, and selection process, but there is only one "common" application. Students complete one application and indicate the undergraduate university or universities for which they wish to be considered. This application is sent directly to NEOMED; a separate undergraduate admissions application to each university is not required. Students in the program are expected to major in "Integrated Life Sciences." The baccalaureate degree will be granted by the participating undergraduate school, while the MD degree will be granted by the NEOMED.

Program Title	The BS / MD Program
Length of Program	6–7 years (two to three undergraduate years)
Number of Students	35
High School Requirements	Minimum SAT of 1210 (combined critical reading and math) or ACT 27 (in place of SAT I score) High school rank/GPA of 3.5 (unweighted)
Application Deadline	December 15
MCAT Requirements	None

Undergraduate Institution: Case Western Reserve University
Medical School: Case Western Reserve University School of Medicine

Undergraduate Contact Information: Undergraduate Admissions Case Western Reserve University Wolstein Hall 11318 Bellflower Rd Cleveland, OH 44106 (216) 368-4450 admission@case.edu	*Medical School Contact Information:* Graduate Admissions CWRU School of Medicine 10900 Euclid Avenue Cleveland, OH 44106 (216) 368-2000 casemed-admissions@case.edu
2014–2015 tuition: $42,766	*2014–2015 tuition*: $55,370
http: //case.edu/ugstudies/pre-professional/scholars-program.html	

About the Medical School

The Case Western Reserve University School of Medicine is a private institution situated on the main campus of the university. The average class size is 145 students.

About the Program

The purpose of the Pre-Professional Scholars Program is to provide premedical college students with a greater sense of freedom and choice in the pursuit of their baccalaureate degrees. Pre-Professional Scholars complete their undergraduate years with a sense of security that enables them to follow courses of study that reflect their educational interests rather than concentrating on activities that they perceive as enhancing their chances of admission to medical school.

Students in the program must maintain a certain GPA throughout their undergraduate educations to be promoted to the School of Medicine. Students are not required to take the MCATs. If they choose to do so, they must achieve a minimum score of 34.

Program Title	Pre-Professional Scholars Program in Medicine
Length of Program	8 years
Number of Students	15 to 20 students
High School Requirements	SAT/ACT and High School Rank/GPA are required (Enrolled students had average SAT over 1410–1510 (combined critical reading and math) and GPA of 3.6/4.0) Three SAT IIs (one of which has to be writing) Demonstration of strong interpersonal skills and leadership
Application Deadline	December 15
MCAT Requirements	Not required (if taken, a minimum score of 34 must be achieved)

Undergraduate Institution: University of Cincinnati
Medical School: University of Cincinnati College of Medicine

Undergraduate Contact Information:	*Medical School Contact Information:*
Office of Admissions University of Cincinnati PO Box 210091 Cincinnati, OH 45221 (513) 556-1100 admissions@uc.edu	Office of Student Affairs University of Cincinnati College of Medicine Medical Sciences Building, Room E251J 231 Albert Sabin Way PO Box 670552 Cincinnati, OH 45267-0552 (513) 558-5581 hs2md@uc.edu
2014–2015 tuition: $10,784 ($25,816 for nonresidents)	*2014–2015 tuition*: $29,680 ($47,944 for nonresidents)
http: //med.uc.edu/connections	

About the Medical School

The University of Cincinnati College of Medicine is a public institution with an average class size of 160. The College of Medicine has established dual admissions programs with the University of Cincinnati that allow high school students to gain admission to medical school from the start of their undergraduate education.

About the BS-MD Program

The College of Engineering and the College of Medicine have developed a special program for exceptional students interested in degrees in both medicine and engineering. This program is designed for the unique student whose interests include the knowledge and skills acquired in an undergraduate engineering education and the scientific and personal expertise obtained in medical school. The total program takes nine years for engineering majors: four years in the College of Engineering, next, a one-year co-op with a medical or pharmaceutical industry, and then four years in the College of Medicine. For premedical majors, the program takes a total of eight years: four years for undergraduate studies and four in the College of Medicine. The program works closely with the honors college to provide a unique and diverse college experience.

Students in the program must maintain a minimum cumulative GPA of 3.4 and a minimum science GPA of 3.4.

Program Title	Connections Dual Admissions Program
Length of Program	8–9 years (4 undergraduate years and possibly a co-op year).
Number of Students	8
High School Requirements	Preference is given to Ohio residents Minimum SAT score of 1300 (combined critical reading and math) or ACT score of 29 High school rank within top 15 percent
Application Deadline	December 2
MCAT Requirements	Yes

Undergraduate Institution: Kent State University
Medical School: Northeastern Ohio Medical University

Undergraduate Contact Information:	Medical School Contact Information:
Undergraduate Admissions 800 E. Summit Street Kent, OH 44240 (330) 672-3000	Director of Admissions Northeastern Ohio Medical University 4209 State Route 44, PO Box 95 Rootstown, OH 44272 (330) 325-6270 admission@neomed.edu
2011–2012 tuition: $23,396 ($31,356 for nonresidents)	*2014–20515 tuition*: $36,950 ($44,915 for nonresidents)

About the Medical School

Northeastern Ohio Medical University (NEOMED) is a public institution dedicated to primary care. The medical school maintains its preclinical campus in Rootstown, Ohio. Clinical training occurs in sixteen local community hospitals. The average class size is 130 students, 105 of which are from the three BS/MD programs sponsored by Northeastern Ohio Medical University

About the Program

The program is designed to allow motivated and bright students the opportunity to complete their premedical and medical educations in less time (either six or seven years with two to three being the undergraduate years) without the stress of medical school admissions. Northeastern Ohio Medical University (NEOMED) offers this program with three undergraduate universities (the University of Akron, Kent State University, and Youngstown State University), which are all within a thirty-five-mile radius of the medical school. The program is open to all students, but preference is given to Ohio residents. Each university has its own BS/MD admissions committee, interviews, and selection process, but there is only one "common" application. Students complete one application and indicate the undergraduate university or universities for which they wish to be considered. This application is sent directly to NEOMED; a separate undergraduate admissions application to each university is not required. Students in the program are expected to major in "Integrated Life Sciences." The baccalaureate degree will be granted by the participating undergraduate school, while the MD degree will be granted by the NEOMED.

Program Title	The BS / MD Program
Length of Program	6–7 years (2–3 undergraduate years)
Number of Students	35
High School Requirements	Preference is given to Ohio residents Minimum SAT 1210 (combined critical reading and math) or ACT of 27 High school rank/GPA of 3.6 (unweighted)
Application Deadline	December 15
MCAT Requirements	None

Undergraduate Institution: University of Miami
Medical School: University of Miami: Miller School of Medicine

Undergraduate Contact Information:	*Medical School Contact Information*:
Office of Undergraduate Admissions University of Miami PO Box 248025 Coral Gables, FL 33124 (305) 384-4323	University of Miami Miller School of Medicine Office of Admissions PO Box 016159 (R-159) Miami, FL 33101–6960 (305) 243-3234 med.admissions@miami.edu
2014–2015 tuition: $21,520	*2011–2012 tuition*: $33,017
http: //www.miami.edu/admission/index.php/ undergraduate_admission/academics/dual_degree_honors	

About the Medical School

The University of Miami School of Medicine is a private institution and is the largest and oldest medical school in Florida. It was founded in 1952. The School of Medicine is located on the medical campus next to Jackson Memorial Hospital in the Civic Center area of Miami. The average class size is 150 students.

About the Program

This program was developed to offer high school students a special opportunity to pursue a broad and enriching education at the undergraduate level. Students will take the usual premedical coursework, and they will also expand their academic and personal experiences to further prepare them to become the physicians of tomorrow. The goals of the program are to develop critical thinking skills, introduce them to health care environments, provide an orientation to medical school coursework, and develop the skills necessary to succeed in demanding medical school environments. Students should enter medical school with greater confidence and a greater level of comfort and maturity.

Students in the program must maintain a minimum cumulative GPA of 3.4 and a minimum science GPA of 3.4. In addition, students are required to take the MCAT during the spring of their junior year.

Program Title	High School Dual Admissions Program
Length of Program	7 or 8 years (3–4 undergraduate years)
High School Requirements	Preference is given to Ohio residents. Minimum SAT score of 1400 (critical reading or math) or ACT score of 32 Minimum SAT II score of 600 in math and one science (chemistry, biology, or physics) High school rank/GPA of 3.75 (unweighted)
Application Deadline	November 1

MCAT Requirements	Yes (minimum score is 27, with a minimum score of 9 or above in Biological Sciences, and no less than an 8 on any other section)

Undergraduate Institution: Youngstown State University
Medical School: Northeastern Ohio Medical University

Undergraduate Contact Information: Office of Admissions Sweeney Welcome Center 1 University Plaza Youngstown, OH 44555	*Medical School Contact Information*: Director of Admissions Northeastern Ohio Medical University 4209 State Route 44, PO Box 95 Rootstown, OH 44272 (330) 325-6270 admission@neomed.edu
2014–2015 tuition: $7,712 ($13,669 for nonresidents)	*2014–2015 tuition*: $36,950 ($44,915 for nonresidents)
http: //www.neomed.edu/admissions/medicine/bsmd	

About the Medical School

Northeastern Ohio Medical University (NEOMED) is a public institution dedicated to primary care. The medical school maintains its preclinical campus in Rootstown, Ohio. Clinical training occurs in sixteen local community hospitals. The average class size is 130 students, 105 of which are from the three BS/MD programs sponsored by Northeastern Ohio Medical University

About the Program

The program is designed to allow motivated and bright students the opportunity to complete their premedical and medical educations in less time (either six or seven years with two to three being the undergraduate years) without the stress of medical school admissions. Northeastern Ohio Medical University (NEOMED) offers this program with three undergraduate universities (the University of Akron, Kent State University, and Youngstown State University), which are all within a thirty-five-mile radius of the medical school. The program is open to all students, but preference is given to Ohio residents. Each university has its own BS/MD admissions committee, interviews, and selection process, but there is only one "common" application. Students complete one application and indicate the undergraduate university or universities for which they wish to be considered. This application is sent directly to NEOMED; a separate undergraduate admissions application to each university is not required. Students in the program are expected to major in "Integrated Life Sciences." The baccalaureate degree will be granted by the participating undergraduate school, while the MD degree will be granted by the NEOMED.

Program Title	The BS/MD Program
Length of Program	6–7 years (2–3 undergraduate years)
Number of Students	35
High School Requirements	Preference is given to Ohio residents SAT/ACT and High School Rank/GPA are required
Application Deadline	December 15
MCAT Requirements	None

Undergraduate Institution: Drexel University
Medical School: Drexel University College of Medicine

Undergraduate Contact Information:	Medical School Contact Information:
Admissions Visit Center Main Building, Room 212, 2nd Floor 3141 Chestnut Street Philadelphia, PA 19104 (215) 895-2400	Admissions Office Drexel School of Medicine 2900 Queen Lane Philadelphia, PA 19129 (215) 991-8202 medadmis@drexel.edu
2014–2015 tuition: $44,646	*2014–2015 tuition*: $51,616
http: //drexel.edu/undergrad/apply/ freshmen-instructions/accelerated/	

About the Medical School

Drexel University College of Medicine is one of the four schools that comprise Drexel University, a private, freestanding academic institution. The Drexel University College of Medicine is the product of the union of two old and well-regarded institutions: the Medical College of Pennsylvania (MCP) founded in 1850 as the first medical school for women, which later became coeducational in 1969, and Hahnemann University, which was founded in 1848 as a private, nondenominational institution. The average class size is 220 students.

About the Program

This program is designed to give talented high school students committed to careers in medicine the opportunity to obtain their educations with less time and lower costs. Students spend two to three years to complete the premedical requirements before being promoted to Drexel University College of Medicine. Students must maintain a minimum of a 3.5 GPA in all coursework throughout their premedical courses. They must also take the MCAT the spring prior to entering medical school.

Program Title	BA/BS/MD Accelerated Degree Program
Length of Program	7–8 years (3–4 undergraduate years)
Number of Students	10
High School Requirements	Minimum SAT score of 1360 (combined critical reading and math) or minimum ACT score of 31 Minimum GPA of 3.5 (unweighted) High school rank within the top 10 percent, minimum recommended Demonstration of strong motivation toward science
Application Deadline	December 1
MCAT Requirements	Yes (must achieve minimum of 9 on verbal and 10 on sciences, or 31 in total—with no section being less than 8)

Undergraduate Institution: Lehigh University
Medical School: Drexel University College of Medicine

Undergraduate Contact Information:	*Medical School Contact Information*:
Office of Admissions Lehigh University 27 Memorial Drive West Bethlehem, PA 18105 (610) 758-3100 cjm2@lehigh.edu	Admissions Office Drexel School of Medicine 2900 Queen Lane Philadelphia, PA 19129 (215) 991-8202 medadmis@drexel.edu
2014–2015 tuition: $44,520	*2014–2015 tuition*: $51,616
http: //www.lehigh.edu/~inbios/ugrad/combined.htm#medicine	

About the Medical School

Drexel University College of Medicine is one of the four schools that comprise Drexel University, a private, freestanding academic institution. The Drexel University College of Medicine is the product of the union of two old and well-regarded institutions: the Medical College of Pennsylvania (MCP) founded in 1850 as the first medical school for women, which later became coeducational in 1969, and Hahnemann University, which was founded in 1848 as a private, nondenominational institution. The average class size is 220 students.

About the Program

This program is designed to give talented high schools students committed to careers in medicine the opportunity to obtain a liberal arts and medical education while reducing the time and cost of their total education.

Students have three years to complete 121 credit hours, before being promoted to Drexel University College of Medicine. Students must maintain a cumulative GPA of 3.45 and take the MCAT the spring before proceeding to medical school. A BA degree in premedical sciences is awarded after the first year of medical school by Lehigh University. The MD will be awarded by Drexel University College of Medicine upon completion of the program.

Program Title	Combined Degree Fast-Track Program in Medicine
Length of Program	7 years (3 undergraduate years)
Number of Students	10
High School Requirements	Minimum SAT Score of 1360 (combined critical reading/math) High school rank within the top 10 percent (minimum recommended)
Application Deadline	November 15

MCAT Requirements	Yes (must achieve minimum of 9 on verbal, 10 on sciences, or 31 in total with no section being less than 8)

Undergraduate Institution: Monmouth University
Medical School: Drexel University College of Medicine

Undergraduate Contact Information: Office of Undergraduate Admissions Monmouth University 400 Cedar Avenue Long Branch, NJ 07764 (732) 571-3400	Medical School Contact Information: Admissions Office Drexel School of Medicine 2900 Queen Lane Philadelphia, PA 19129 (215) 991-8202 medadmis@drexel.edu
2014–2015 tuition: $16,355	*2014–2015 tuition*: $51,616
http: //www.monmouth.edu/academics/pre-professional_health/medical_scholars.asp	

About the Medical School

Drexel University College of Medicine is one of the four schools that comprise Drexel University, a private, freestanding academic institution. The Drexel University College of Medicine is the product of the union of two old and well-regarded institutions: the Medical College of Pennsylvania (MCP) founded in 1850 as the first medical school for women, which later became coeducational in 1969, and Hahnemann University, which was founded in 1848 as a private, nondenominational institution. The average class size is 220 students.

About the Program

The Monmouth Medical Center Scholars Program is directed toward students who have excelled academically and who wish to enter the medical disciplines of family medicine, general internal medicine, or general pediatrics.

Students must maintain a cumulative minimum GPA of 3.3 while at Monmouth and take the MCAT during their junior year. Students spend a one-semester preceptorship at the Monmouth Medical Center during their senior year at Monmouth University.

Program Title	The Monmouth Medical Center Scholars Program
Length of Program	8 years
Number of Students	4
High School Requirements	New Jersey residents only Minimum SAT score of 1270 (combined critical reading and math) with no score below 560 GPA of 3.5 out of 4.0 (minimum) Demonstration of interest in primary care
Application Deadline	December 1
MCAT Requirements	Yes (must achieve a minimum score of 9 on the verbal, 10 or better on sciences, or a total of 31 with no score less than 8)

Undergraduate Institution: Pennsylvania State University
Medical School: Sidney Kimmel Medical College of Thomas Jefferson University

Undergraduate Contact Information:	*Medical School Contact Information:*
Undergraduate Admissions Office Pennsylvania State University 201 Shields Building Box 3000 University Park, PA 16804 (814) 865-5471	Associate Dean for Admissions Jefferson Medical College 1015 Walnut Street, Suit 110 Philadelphia, PA 19107 (215) 955-6983 SKMC.Admissions@ jefferson.edu

2014–2015 tuition: $16,572 ($29,522 for nonresidents)	2014–2015 tuition: $52,266
http: //science.psu.edu/premed/premedmed/ accelerated-premed-medical	

About the Medical School

Founded in 1824, Jefferson Medical College has conferred more than 27,000 medical degrees and has more living graduates than any other medical school in the nation. It offers both undergraduate medical education programs and innovative joint health degree programs to more than 1,000 students each year.

About the Program

The Premedical-Medical Accelerated Program began in 1963 as an agreement between Pennsylvania State College of Science and the Jefferson Medical College. Students can earn the BS and MD degrees in six years (four summers make one term) or seven years (with summers off).

Students spend the first two or three years at Penn State University in State College and then proceed to medical school for its regular four-year curriculum. The BS is awarded after the first or second year in medical school, depending on whether the student selected the six or seven year program.

Program Title	Accelerated Premedical-Medical Program
Length of Program	6 or 7 years (2–3 undergraduate years)
Number of Students	25
High School Requirements	Minimum SAT score of 2100 or ACT score of 32 Top 10 percent of the class
Application Deadline	November 30
MCAT Requirements	Yes (must achieve a minimum score of 30 with no subset less than 9)

Undergraduate Institution: Rosemont College
Medical School: Drexel University College of Medicine

Undergraduate Contact Information:	*Medical School Contact Information:*
Health Professions Adviser	Admissions Office
Department of Biology	Drexel School of Medicine
Rosemont College	2900 Queen Lane
1400 Montgomery Avenue	Philadelphia, PA 19129
Rosemont, PA 19010	(215) 991-8202
(610) 527-0200	medadmis@drexel.edu
jsquire@rosemont.edu	
2014–2015 tuition: $31,580	*2014–2015 tuition*: $51,616
http: //www.rosemont.edu/academics/undergraduate/ special-programs/collaborative-programs.php	

About the Medical School

Drexel University College of Medicine is one of the four schools that comprise Drexel University, a private, freestanding academic institution. The Drexel University College of Medicine is the product of the union of two old and well-regarded institutions: the Medical College of Pennsylvania (MCP) founded in 1850 as the first medical school for women, which later became coeducational in 1969, and Hahnemann University, which was founded in 1848 as a private, nondenominational institution. The average class size is 220 students.

About the Program

The Rosemont Early Assurance Program is intended for academically select and highly motivated high school students who are interested in careers in medicine. It assures the students meeting the standards of the program admission to the medical school after their senior year at Rosemont.

Students in the program must maintain a cumulative minimum GPA of 3.5, especially a science GPA of 3.25. Students must take the MCAT in the spring of their junior year.

Program Title	Early Assurance Program
Length of Program	8 years
Number of Students	4
High School Requirements	Minimum SAT score of 1300 (combined critical reading and math with at least a 600 on each section) or ACT score of 29 Minimum GPA 3.5 (unweighted) High school rank within top 10 percent
Application Deadline	December 1
MCAT Requirements	Yes (must achieve a minimum score of 31)

Undergraduate Institution: Temple University
Medical School: Temple University School of Medicine

Undergraduate Contact Information:	Medical School Contact Information:
Health Professions Advising Center Temple University 1810 Liacouras Walk, Suite 100 Philadelphia, PA, 19122 (215) 204-2513 healthadvising@temple.edu	Office of Admissions Temple University School of Medicine 3500 N. Broad Street Philadelphia, PA 19140 (215) 707-3656 medadmissions@temple.edu
2014–2015 tuition: $14,696 ($24,722 for nonresidents)	2014–2015 tuition: $44,344 ($54,158 for nonresidents)
http: //www.temple.edu/healthadvising/healthscholars.html	

About the Medical School

Temple University School of Medicine (TUSOM) is a public institution that opened in 1901. The School of Medicine prioritizes three things: education, research, and the clinical care of all, including the most impoverished. The average class size is 210 students.

About the Program

The Pre-Med Health Scholar Program provides an opportunity for outstanding students to gain conditional admission to the Temple University School of Medicine at the same time they are accepted into one of Temple's undergraduate colleges. As a Pre-Med Health Scholar, students spend their undergraduate years in Temple's Honor Program, after which they will enroll into Temple University School of Medicine, leading to the doctor of medicine degree. The program was made for students with impressive high school records who have demonstrated an interest in the field of medicine.

Students in the program must maintain a 3.5 cumulative and science GPA and take the MCAT the spring of their junior year. Students must also gain exposure in the health care professions by volunteering, community service, and research.

Program Title	Pre-Med Health Scholar Program
Length of Program	7–8 years (3–4 undergraduate years)
Number of Students	10
High School Requirements	Minimum SAT score of 1350 (combined critical reading and math) or ACT score of 32 Minimum GPA of 3.8 (unweighted) Demonstrated commitment to service/ volunteer opportunities
Application Deadline	January 14
MCAT Requirements	Yes (must achieve a minimum score of 30, with no section less than 9)

Undergraduate Institution: University of Pittsburgh
Medical School: University of Pittsburgh School of Medicine

Undergraduate Contact Information: University of Pittsburgh Office of Admissions and Financial Aid Alumni Hall, 4227 Fifth Avenue Pittsburgh, PA 15260-6601 (412) 624–PITT (7488) oafa@pitt.edu	*Medical School Contact Information:* University of Pittsburgh School of Medicine Office of Admissions and Financial Aid 518 Scaife Hall 3550 Terrace Street Pittsburgh, PA 15261 (412) 648-9891 admissions@medschool.pitt.edu
2014–2015 tuition: $16,872 ($27,268 for nonresidents)	*2014–2015 tuition*: $48,792 ($50,014 for nonresidents)
http: //www.medadmissions.pitt.edu/admissions-requirements/guaranteed-admissions.php	

About the Medical School

The University of Pittsburgh School of Medicine is a public institution founded in 1886. The goal of the School of Medicine is to educate physicians who are prepared to meet the challenges of practicing medicine and conducting cutting-edge biomedical research focused on bettering the human condition. The average class size is 148 students.

About the Program

The Guaranteed Admissions Program is designed to allow early admission to medical school for those students interested in bioengineering as well as medicine. This program permits students to major in bioengineering during their undergraduate years and then continue to medical school.

Students in the program must maintain a minimum cumulative and science GPA of 3.75. It is not required for students to take the MCAT in this program.

Program Title	Guaranteed Admissions Program
Length of Program	8 years
High School Requirements	Minimum SAT score of 1450 (combined critical reading and math) or ACT score of 33 High school rank within top 10 percent
Application Deadline	December 1
MCAT Requirements	Not required

Undergraduate Institution: Ursinus College
Medical School: Drexel University College of Medicine

Undergraduate Contact Information: Office of Admissions Ursinus College 601 E. Main Street Collegeville, PA 19426-1000 (610) 409-3200 admission@ursinus.edu	Medical School Contact Information: Admissions Office Drexel School of Medicine 2900 Queen Lane Philadelphia, PA 19129 (215) 991-8202 medadmis@drexel.edu
2014–2015 tuition: $45,890	2014–2015 tuition: $51,616
http: //www.ursinus.edu/netcommunity/page.aspx?pid=440	

About the Medical School

Drexel University College of Medicine is one of the four schools that comprise Drexel University, a private, freestanding academic institution. The Drexel University College of Medicine is the product of the union of two old and well-regarded institutions: the Medical College of Pennsylvania (MCP) founded in 1850 as the first medical school for women, which later became coeducational in 1969, and Hahnemann

University, which was founded in 1848 as a private, nondenominational institution. The average class size is 220 students.

About the Program

The Early Assurance Program is intended for academically select and highly motivated high school students interested in medical careers. It assures students meeting the standards of the program admission to medical school after their senior year at Ursinus College. This program also offers students an added degree of freedom to explore other interests and courses in the liberal arts.

Students in the program must maintain a cumulative and science minimum GPA of 3.5, and take the MCAT in the spring of their junior year.

Program Title	Ursinus/Drexel Early Assurance Program
Length of Program	8 years
Number of Students	4
High School Requirements	Minimum SAT score of 1300 (combined critical reading and math with no subset less that 560) High school rank within top 10 percent Strong commitment to medicine and medical experience
Application Deadline	November 15
MCAT Requirements	Yes (must achieve a minimum of 9 on verbal and 10 on sciences or a 31 with no score less than 8) Must also attain an "M" on the writing section

Undergraduate Institution: Villanova University
Medical School: Drexel University College of Medicine

103

Undergraduate Contact Information:	*Medical School Contact Information:*
Office of University Admission	Admissions Office
Villanova University	Drexel School of Medicine
Austin Hall	2900 Queen Lane
800 Lancaster Avenue	Philadelphia, PA 19129
Villanova, PA 19085–1699	(215) 991-8202
(610) 519-4833	medadmis@drexel.edu
hpa@villanova.edu	
2014–2015 tuition: $45,376	*2014–2015 tuition*: $51,616
http: //www1.villanova.edu/villanova/artsci/undergrad/ resources/health/affiliates/medicine.html	

About the Medical School

Drexel University College of Medicine is one of the four schools that comprise Drexel University, a private, freestanding academic institution. The Drexel University College of Medicine is the product of the union of two old and well-regarded institutions: the Medical College of Pennsylvania (MCP) founded in 1850 as the first medical school for women, which later became coeducational in 1969, and Hahnemann University, which was founded in 1848 as a private, nondenominational institution. The average class size is 220 students.

About the Program

This program is designed to give talented high schools students committed to careers in medicine the opportunity to obtain their education with less time and lower cost.

Students can spend two or three years at Villanova before being promoted to Drexel University College of Medicine. Students must maintain a cumulative and science GPA of 3.5 and take the MCAT the spring before proceeding to medical school.

Program Title	Fast Track BS/MD Program
Length of Program	6–7 years (2–3 undergraduate years).
Number of Students	10
High School Requirements	Minimum SAT score of 1360 (combined critical reading and math—with no subset less than 600) or ACT score of 31 Minimum GPA of 3.8 (unweighted) High school rank within the top 5 percent Demonstration of exposure to hospital settings
Application Deadline	November 1
MCAT Requirements	Yes (must achieve a 9 minimum on the verbal with a 10 on each section of the sciences or a 31 total with no section less than 8)

Undergraduate Institution: West Chester University
Medical School: Drexel University College of Medicine

Undergraduate Contact Information:	Medical School Contact Information:
Office of Undergraduate Admissions West Chester University 100 West Rosedale Avenue West Chester, PA 19393 (610) 436-3411 ugadmiss@wcupa.edu	Admissions Office Drexel School of Medicine 2900 Queen Lane Philadelphia, PA 19129 (215) 991-8202 medadmis@drexel.edu
2014–2015 tuition: $9,144 ($19,592 for nonresidents)	2014–2015 tuition: $51,616
http: //www.wcupa.edu/_ACADEMICS/ SCH_CAS/MED/Early_Assurance_Undergrad/pdf/ DEA_Standards_Instructions_Checklist.pdf	

About the Medical School

Drexel University College of Medicine is one of the four schools that comprise Drexel University, a private, freestanding academic institution. The Drexel University College of Medicine is the product of the union of two old and well-regarded institutions: the Medical College of Pennsylvania (MCP) founded in 1850 as the first medical school for women, which later became coeducational in 1969, and Hahnemann University, which was founded in 1848 as a private, nondenominational institution. The average class size is 220 students.

About the BS-MD Program

This cooperative program is intended for the academically select and highly motivated high school students who are interested in medical careers. It assures the accepted student meeting the standards of the program admission to the Drexel University College of Medicine after their senior year at West Chester University.

Students in the program must maintain a cumulative and science minimum GPA of 3.5 and take the MCAT exam in the spring of their junior year.

Program Title	West Chester/Drexel Early Assurance Program
Length of Program	8 years
Number of Students	6
High School Requirements	Minimum SAT score of 1300 (combined critical reading and math with no section less that 560) High school rank within the top 10 percent Minimum GPA of 3.5 (unweighted)
Application Deadline	November 15

MCAT Requirements	Yes (must achieve minimum of 9 on verbal and 10 on science sections or 31 total with no section less than 8)

Undergraduate Institution: Widener University
Medical School: Temple University School of Medicine

Undergraduate Contact Information: Pre-Medical Program Adviser Widener University One University Place Chester, PA 19013 (610) 499-4020 aanagengast@mail.weidner.edu	*Medical School Contact Information:* Office of Admissions Temple University School of Medicine 3500 N. Broad Street Philadelphia, PA 19140 (215) 707-3656 medadmissions@temple.edu
2014–2015 tuition: $39,052	*2014–2015 tuition*: $44,344 ($54,158 for nonresidents)
http: //www.widener.edu/academics/schools/arts_sciences/ sciences/premed/medical_scholars.aspx	

About the Medical School

Temple University School of Medicine (TUSOM) is a public institution that opened in 1901. The School of Medicine prioritizes three things: education, research, and the clinical care of all including the most impoverished. The average class size is 210 students.

About the Program

The Widener Medical Scholars Program offers early assurance admission to Temple University School of Medicine for highly qualified high school seniors. The program has been designed to attract broadly educated candidates who are interested in entering the practice of primary care medicine, general internal medicine, or general pediatrics. Once selected for the program, students participate in a well-integrated undergraduate and medical experience that involves a variety of experiences at the local Crozer-Chester Medical Center.

Students in the program may choose any major at Widener. Students must maintain a cumulative GPA of 3.3 and take the MCAT in the spring of their junior year.

Program Title	The Widener Medical Scholars Program
Length of Program	8 years
Number of Students	8
High School Requirements	Must be a resident of Pennsylvania, Delaware, New Jersey, or Maryland Minimum SAT score of 1350 (combined critical reading and math) with none of the three sections lower than 600
Application Deadline	October 4
MCAT Requirements	Yes (minimum scores not defined)

Undergraduate Institution: Wilkes University
Medical School: State University of New York—Upstate Medical University

Undergraduate Contact Information:	Medical School Contact Information:
Health Sciences Adviser Department of Biology, Chemistry & Health Sciences Wilkes University 84 West South Street Wilkes-Barre, PA 18766 (570) 408-4400 admissions@wilkes.edu	Student Admissions SUNY Upstate 1215 Weiskotten Hall 766 Irving Avenue Syracuse, New York 13210 (315) 464-4570 admiss@upstate.edu

2014–2015 tuition: $31,262	2014–2015 tuition: $27,090 ($53,650 for nonresidents)
http: //bulletin.wilkes.edu/7430.htm	

About the Medical School

State University of New York—Upstate Medical University (SUNY Upstate) began in 1835 and initially started as the Geneva Medical College (GMC). SUNY Upstate is known for its research, clinical, and biotechnological facilities

About the Program

The Premedical Scholars Program is designed to allow early admission to medical school for those students with an interest in pursuing careers as physicians. The program selects talented high school students from the southern tier of New York.

Students in the program must maintain a cumulative minimum GPA of 3.3 and a science GPA of 3.5. Students must take the MCAT during the spring of their junior year. Students also spend one semester at the Robert Packer Hospital at the Guthrie Clinic, conducting clinical and basic science research. During the third and fourth years of medical school, the students are required to do clinical rotations at the Robert Packer Hospital at the Guthrie Clinic.

Program Title	Premedical Scholars Program
Length of Program	8 years
Number of Students	6
High School Requirements	Only residents from the southern tier of New York (from Binghamton to Elmira/Corning) Minimum SAT score of 1200 (combined critical reading and math)
Application Deadline	November 15
MCAT Requirements	Yes (minimum score not specified)

Undergraduate Institution: Wilkes University
Medical School: Pennsylvania State University College of Medicine

Undergraduate Contact Information:	Medical School Contact Information:
Health Sciences Adviser Department of Biology, Chemistry & Health Sciences Wilkes University 84 West South Street Wilkes-Barre, PA 18766 (570) 408-4400 admissions@wilkes.edu	Office of Student Affairs Penn State College of Medicine 500 University Drive, H060 Hershey, PA 17033 (717) 531-8755
2014–2015 tuition: $31,262	*2014–2015 tuition*: $41,860 ($52,146 for nonresidents)
http: //bulletin.wilkes.edu/7428.htm	

About the Medical School

The Penn State College of Medicine is a public institution founded in 1963. The College of Medicine was a joint venture between the Milton S. Hershey Foundation and Pennsylvania State University. The average class size is 110 students.

About the Program

The Premedical Scholars Program with the Penn State College of Medicine is designed to allow early admission to medical school for those students from rural and medically underserved areas of Pennsylvania who have a sincere interest in pursuing careers as primary care physicians.

Students in the program must maintain a minimum cumulative and science GPA of 3.5 and take the MCAT during the spring of their junior year. Students also spend one semester at the Robert Packer Hospital of the Guthrie Clinic or the Wilkes-Barre General Hospital. During the third and fourth years at medical school, students are required to do clinical rotations at either the Robert Packer Hospital of the Guthrie Clinic or at the Wilkes-Barre General Hospital.

Program Title	Premedical Scholars Program with Penn State
Length of Program	8 years
Number of Students	2
High School Requirements	Must be a Pennsylvania rural or medically underserved area Minimum SAT score of 1250 (critical reading and math) High school rank within the top 10 percent
Application Deadline	November 15
MCAT Requirements	Yes (must achieve at least the national average)

Undergraduate Institution: Brown University
Medical School: Warren Alpert Medical School of Brown University

Undergraduate Contact Information:	*Medical School Contact Information:*
College Admissions Office Brown University Box 1876 Providence, RI 02912 (401) 863-2378 admission@brown.edu	Office of Admissions Warren Alpert medical school of Brown University 222 Richmond Street, 1ˢᵗ Floor Providence, RI 02912 (401) 863-2149 MedSchool_Admissions@ brown.edu
2014–2015 tuition: $46,408	*2014–2015 tuition*: $47,480
http: //www.brown.edu/academics/medical/plme/	

About the Medical School

Brown University is a private institution founded in 1764. The Brown University School of Medicine was established in 1975. The School of Medicine only accepts individuals applying for the MD-PhD program into the first-year class unless they are enrolled in specific postbaccalaureate programs, early-admissions programs, or are a Brown University undergraduate student. The majority of the School of Medicine is comprised of students in the Program in Liberal Medical Education. The average class size is seventy.

About the Program

Brown's Program in Liberal Medical Education offers a unique opportunity to combine undergraduate and professional studies in medicine in an eight-year continuum. The program combines the open curriculum concept of the undergraduate school and the competency-based curriculum concept of the medical school. It encourages students interested in medicine to pursue other interests (humanities, social sciences, natural sciences, etc.) in depth as they prepare for careers as physicians. While the program usually takes eight years, the students can take part of the Flex Plan. The Flex Plan defers entry to medical school by one or two more years to pursue other interests like education, research, public service, government, health care, and business.

Program Title	The Program in Liberal Medical Education
Length of Program	8 years
Number of Students	50
High School Requirements	SAT I test and two SAT II tests (one being a science subject test) or the ACT test (minimum not defined) Enrolled students in top 2 percent on class
Application Deadline	January 1
MCAT Requirements	None

Undergraduate Institution: Rice University
Medical School: Baylor College of Medicine

Undergraduate Contact Information:	Medical School Contact Information:
Office of Admissions—MS-17 Rice University 6100 Main Street Houston, TX 77005 (713) 348-7423 admi@rice.edu	Office of Admissions Baylor College of Medicine One Baylor Plaza Houston, TX 77030 (713) 798-4842 admissions@bcm.edu
2014–2015 tuition: $39,880	2014–2015 tuition: $26,966 ($40,066 for nonresidents)
http: //futureowls.rice.edu/futureowls/Medical_Scholars.asp	

About the Medical School

The Baylor College of Medicine is a private institution and is the academic center of the Texas Medical Center in Houston. The college has several education outreach programs that start as early as kindergarten to cultivate the passion for medicine and science. The school emphasizes the need to be continuous learners and striving to always learn. The average class size is 170 students.

About the Program

The Medical Scholars Program promotes the education of future physicians who are scientifically competent, compassionate, and socially conscious. The program provides selected students with the opportunity to increase their knowledge and skills without worrying how curricular or extracurricular choices made in college might affect medical school admission. It is the hope of Rice University and Baylor College of Medicine that these students will apply insights from their extensive study of the liberal arts with the study of modern medical science. Thus, accepted students are encouraged to explore the entire range of Rice University undergraduate programs to the extent that their interests allow.

Students in the program must maintain a minimum cumulative GPA of 3.2. They are required to take the MCAT, but a minimum score to achieve is not specified.

Program Title	The Medical Scholars Program
Length of Program	8 years
Number of Students	10
High School Requirements	SAT or ACT scores required SAT II in three subjects required GPA/rank required (enrolled students were within top 5 percent) Shown commitment to the field of medicine
Application Deadline	December 1
MCAT Requirements	Yes (no minimum requirement)

Undergraduate Institution: Texas A&M University
Medical School: Texas A&M University Health Sciences Center College of Medicine

Undergraduate Contact Information:	*Medical School Contact Information:*
Office of Undergraduate Admissions Texas A&M University PO Box 30014 College Station, TX 77842–3014 (979) 845-1060 admissions@tamu.edu	Texas A&M Health Science Center College of Medicine Office of Admissions Health Professions Education Building 8447 Highway 47 Bryan, TX 77807 (979) 436-0237

2014–2015 tuition: $9,180	2014–2015 tuition: $42,961
($26,356 for nonresidents)	($56,061 for nonresidents)
http: //medicine.tamhsc.edu/admissions/ppc/ppc-brochure.pdf	

About the Medical School

The Texas A&M University College of Medicine is a public institution established in 1973 as part of the Texas A&M University Health Science Center. The average class size is 200 students.

About the Program

The Partnership in Primary Care program is designed to offer highly qualified high school students, who are residents of Texas, the opportunity to broaden their educational experiences and explore interdisciplinary programs and projects. This program is specifically designed for students who want to eventually help underserved parts of Texas as primary care physicians. Admission into this program allows the students a range of workshops to participate in during their undergraduate years to help enrich their studies.

To matriculate to medical school, students must maintain a cumulative GPA of 3.50. Students must also take the MCAT and achieve a minimum score of 25 (with no section below 7).

Program Title	Partnership in Primary Care
Length of Program	8 years
Number of Students	15
High School Requirements	Must be a Texas resident
	Minimum GPA of 3.5 (unweighted)
	High school rank in top 10 percent
	Minimum SAT score of 1200 (combined critical reading and math) or ACT score of 26
	Interested in becoming a primary care physician

Application Deadline	February 15
MCAT Requirements	Yes (minimum score of 25 with no section below 7)

Undergraduate Institution: Virginia Commonwealth University
Medical School: Virginia Commonwealth University School of Medicine

Undergraduate Contact Information:	*Medical School Contact Information*:
The Honors College Virginia Commonwealth University 701 West Grace Street PO Box 843010 Richmond, Virginia 23284 (804) 828-1803 stuacctg@vcu.edu	Office of Admissions VCU School of Medicine McGlothlin Medical Education Center 1201 E. Marshall St., 1st Floor PO Box 980565 Richmond, VA 23298 (804) 828-9629 somume@vcu.edu
2013–2014 tuition: $12,002 ($28,861 for nonresidents)	*2014–2015 tuition*: $29,091 ($44,443 for nonresidents)
https: //www.pubapps.vcu.edu/honors/guaranteed/medicine/index.aspx	

About the Medical School

The Virginia Commonwealth University School of Medicine is a public institution, originally founded in 1838 as the Medical College of Virginia. The School of Medicine is situated in downtown Richmond in the Medical College of Virginia campus, which also houses the other schools of health professions. The average class size is 170 students.

About the Program

The Guaranteed Admission Program offers academically capable and highly focused students an opportunity to pursue intellectually challenging programs of study without the pressure of competing further for medical school admission. Close contact with the School of Medicine throughout the undergraduate program aids students in testing their career choice and in preparing for a lifelong commitment to learning in the profession.

Accepted students will participate in the Honors Program and are required to maintain a minimum cumulative GPA of 3.5 and fulfill all their baccalaureate requirements before promotion to the medical school.

Program Title	Guaranteed Admissions Program in Medicine
Length of Program	8 years
Number of Students	15
High School Requirements	Minimum SAT score of 1910 (with no one score less than 530) or ACT score of 29 Minimum GPA of 3.5 (unweighted) Demonstration of health care–related activities
Application Deadline	November 15
MCAT Requirements	None